Fracture Finder: A Practical Guide to Interpreting Upper and Lower Limb X-Rays for Radiographers

Suman Moughal

Fracture Finder: A Practical Guide to Interpreting Upper and Lower Limb X-Rays for Radiographers

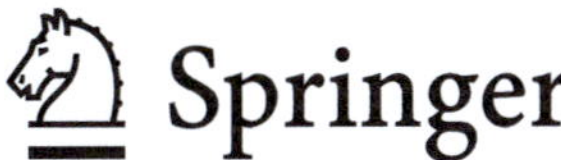

Suman Moughal
Queen Elizabeth Hospital Birmingham
Birmingham, UK

ISBN 978-3-032-17323-2   ISBN 978-3-032-17324-9   (eBook)
https://doi.org/10.1007/978-3-032-17324-9

This Springer imprint is published by the registered company Springer Nature Switzerland AG
The registered company address is: Gewerbestrasse 11, 6330 Cham, Switzerland

If disposing of this product, please recycle the paper.

Preface

Radiography is both an art and a science, demanding precision, knowledge and a deep understanding of anatomy, pathology and patient care. As a qualified specialist radiographer working in a major trauma centre and as a student liaison, I have witnessed first-hand the challenges faced by student radiographers as they transition from the classroom to clinical practice.

This handbook was created to bridge that gap. It is designed to serve as a clear and accessible resource for students and newly qualified radiographers navigating the complexities of trauma imaging and routine examinations. Focused on the most common pathologies and fractures encountered in clinical settings, this guide emphasises practical information, including identifying abnormalities on X-ray images, understanding centring points and recognising the required areas of interest for each examination.

Whether you are studying for exams, preparing for placements or seeking a quick refresher on the job, this book is structured to support your learning with clarity and confidence.

This resource not only enhances your technical understanding but also encourages you to grow in clinical reasoning, image evaluation and patient-centred practice.

Welcome to the start—or continuation—of a rewarding journey in radiography.

Birmingham, UK   Suman Moughal

Fracture Description Guidelines

It can be challenging to remember all the key points when describing an image, especially when pathology is present.

A helpful way to ensure nothing is missed is by using a mnemonic. Here is one you can use to guide your image descriptions:

Let's Focus on Correct Image Detail
L—Location
F—Fracture orientation
O—Open or Closed
C—Comminuted
I—Intra-articular
D—Displacement

- Location
    - Identify the anatomical Area involved (e.g., hand, wrist).
    - Specify the exact location of the pathology, such as the specific bone (e.g., first metacarpal) and the region of the bone affected (e.g., metaphysis, epiphysis).
- Fracture Orientation
    - Describe the direction of the fracture line—e.g., transverse, oblique, spiral or longitudinal.
- Open or Closed
    - Determine whether the fracture is open (bone has broken through the skin) or closed (skin remains intact).
- Comminution
    - Assess whether the fracture is comminuted, meaning the bone is broken into more than two fragments.
- Intra-articular Involvement
    - Note that if the fracture extends into a joint space, it is classified as intra-articular.
- Displacement and Angulation
    - Comment on any displacement (movement of bone fragments from their normal position) and angulation (change in the normal axis of the bone).

Bone Anatomy

The image below (Fig. 1) illustrates the anatomical features of a typical bone, including the diaphysis, metaphysis and epiphysis. The tibia, one of the long bones of the lower leg, is used here as an example.

Types of Fractures

The image below (Fig. 2) illustrates the common types of fracture patterns identifiable on X-rays.

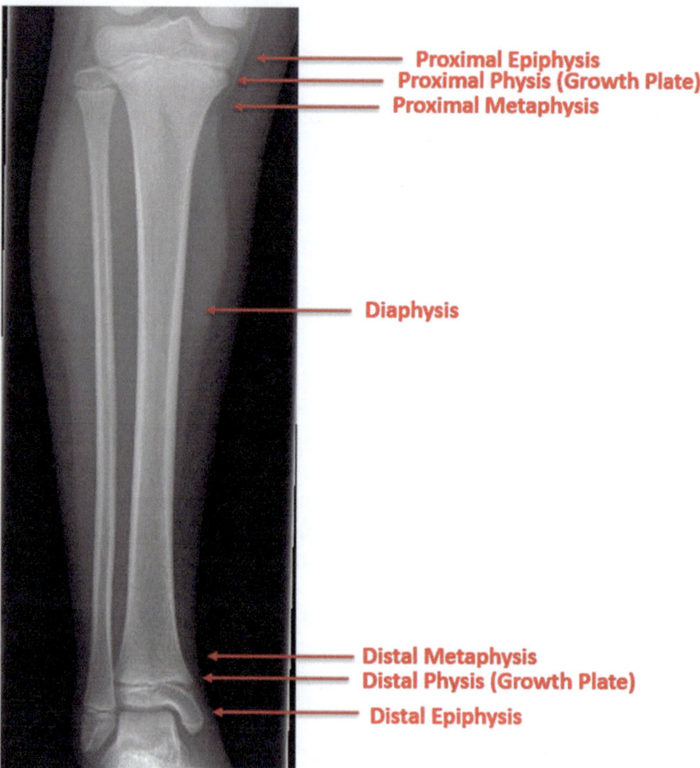

Fig. 1 Anatomical structure of the bone

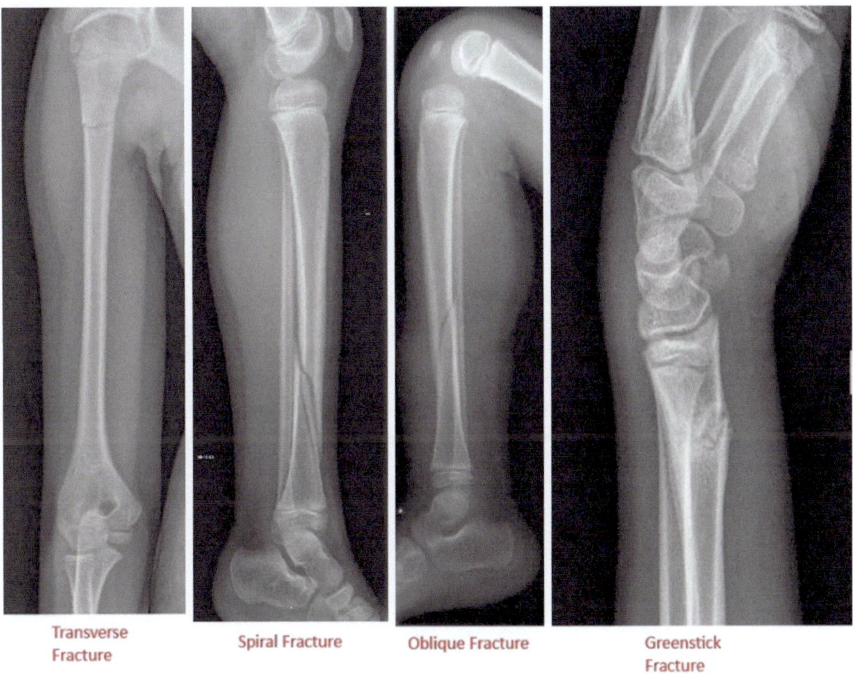

Fig. 2 Different types of fracture orientations

How to Assess Images

1. Projection and Views
   - Have the correct projections been taken for the clinical indication? Ensure that the standard views required for the area examined have been performed to avoid missing any pathology.
   - Is the positioning appropriate for the projection? Has the correct anatomical region been imaged and centred accurately (refer to the specific centring point for the examination)?
   - Have additional views been taken if needed, such as oblique or comparison images, especially in trauma or joint evaluation?
2. Collimation
   - Has the image been collimated appropriately to include the entire area of interest without excluding relevant anatomy?
   - Tight collimation is essential to reduce patient dose and improve image quality by minimising scatter.
3. Image Quality
   - Are the exposure factors appropriate for the body part and patient size? Check that the exposure index (EI) falls within the acceptable range for your specific X-ray equipment.
   - Does the image appear too light or too dark? Assess the overall brightness and density—you should visualise the trabecular bone pattern and surrounding soft tissues.
   - Is there adequate contrast to differentiate between bone, soft tissue, and air? Poor contrast can hinder diagnosis.
   - Is the image sharp and well-defined? Blurring may suggest patient movement or incorrect focus-to-film distance.
   - Are there any artefacts (e.g., clothing, jewellery, motion) that obscure the anatomy?
4. Anatomy and Pathology
   - Is the relevant anatomy fully included and demonstrated?
   - Examine for any signs of pathology, such as:
     - Cortical irregularities (e.g., step-offs or angulation indicating fracture)
     - Misalignment or dislocation
     - Degenerative changes
     - Foreign bodies

- Compare with previous images or the opposite side, if available and clinically appropriate.
5. Need for Repeat
   - Based on your evaluation, is the image diagnostically acceptable?
   - If key anatomy is missing, exposure is inadequate, or pathology cannot be confidently ruled out, a repeat image may be necessary—but always justify any additional exposure.

Acknowledgements

I want to express my deepest gratitude to my family and friends for their unwavering support and encouragement throughout this journey. Your belief in me has been a constant source of strength.

Also, a big thank you to my mentor, AJP, from Newcross Hospital, who helped me believe in myself and provided the support and encouragement I needed to complete my three years of training. I am also sincerely grateful to Dr Steve Amerasekera, who supported me in creating this book.

This book is dedicated to all aspiring radiographers and healthcare professionals. May it serve as a practical and empowering resource throughout your clinical journey.

Contents

To accurately comment on, highlight, or identify abnormalities, it is essential to understand the fundamentals, which include being familiar with the standard imaging views and the correct centring points to ensure high-quality diagnostic images.

This chapter will cover the most common pathologies found in the upper limb, including:

    I. Fingers
   II. Hand
  III. Wrist
  IV. Scaphoid
   V. Forearm
  VI. Elbow
 VII. Humerus
VIII. Shoulder
  IX. Clavicle

It will also outline the standard radiographic views and centring points for each area, along with guidance on how to describe the images using the method outlined on page 8.

Fingers 1

Figure 1.1 demonstrates the basic anatomical structures visible on both standard Dorsi-Palmar (DP) and Lateral finger x-rays.

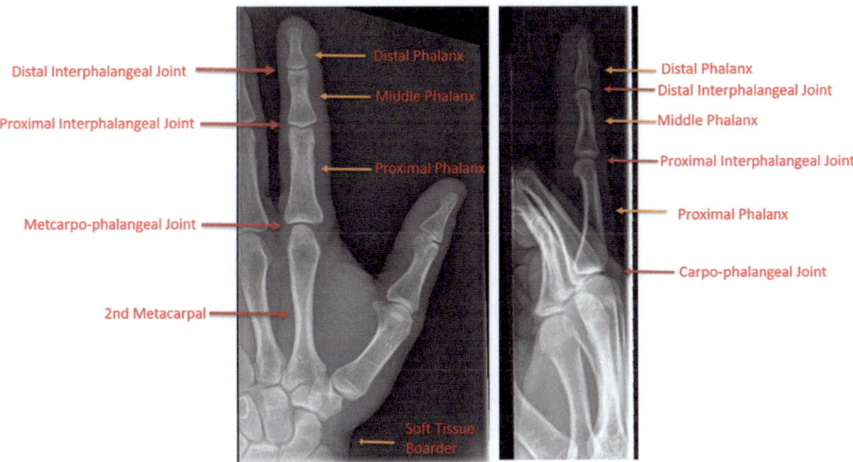

Fig. 1.1 Anatomical structures of the fingers on the DP and Lateral views

© The Author(s), under exclusive license to Springer Nature Switzerland AG 2026
S. Moughal, *Fracture Finder: A Practical Guide to Interpreting Upper and Lower Limb X-Rays for Radiographers*,
https://doi.org/10.1007/978-3-032-17324-9_1

1.1   Standard Views, Centring Points and Area of Interest

Dorsi Palmar The hand is placed on the image receptor with the palmar aspect on the image receptor. The affected finger should be fully extended, with the centring point being over the proximal interphalangeal joint.

Lateral The hand is placed in the centre of the image receptor with the lateral aspect in contact with the image receptor. The affected finger should be extended, while the non-affected fingers should be flexed to ensure they are not in the field of view. The centring point is over the proximal interphalangeal joint of the affected finger.

Area of Interest In both views, the distal end of the metacarpal to the fingertip should be visualised, including the surrounding soft tissue [1].

1.2   General Evaluation of Finger Examinations

1. The area of interest must be included, from the distal phalanx to the metacarpophalangeal (MCP) joint.
2. Adjacent soft tissues and surrounding fingers should be visible to assess for swelling, foreign bodies or soft tissue injury.
3. No rotation unless intentional (e.g., oblique view).
4. Clear visualisation of bone trabeculae and cortical outlines, indicating correct exposure factors.
5. Joints (distal interphalangeal (DIP), proximal interphalangeal (PIP) and metacarpal phalangeal (MCP) should be open and clearly defined if positioning is optimal.
6. The finger should be lined up straight with the image receptor.

1.3   Common Finger Fractures/Pathologies

1.3.1   Volar Plate Avulsion Fracture

This is a small fracture fragment, known as an avulsion fracture, seen on the palmar (volar) aspect of the base of the middle phalanx. This is represented in the image below (Fig. 1.2).

1.3.2   Extensor Tendon Avulsion Fracture

An Avulsion Fracture is located on the dorsal aspect of the base of the distal phalanx. This type of fracture can be associated with mallet finger injuries (described on page 17), where the tendon may pull a small piece of bone away from its attachment.
    This fracture is represented in Fig. 1.3.

Fig. 1.2 Volar plate avulsion fracture at the base of the middle phalanx

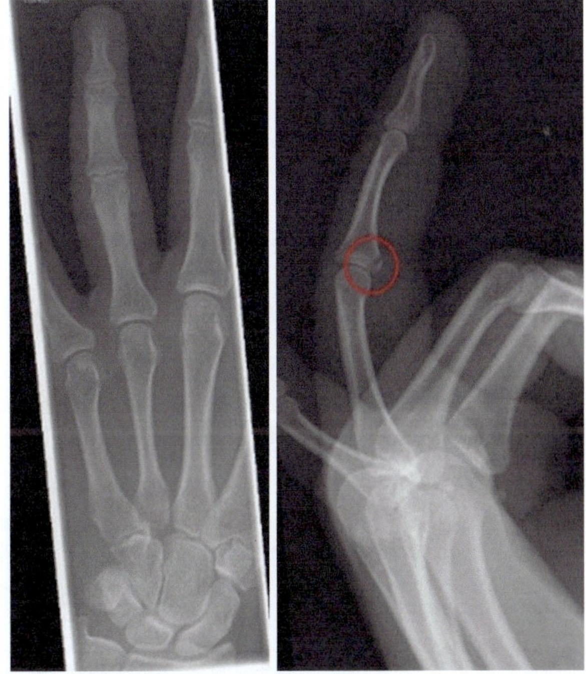

Fig. 1.3 Extensor tendon avulsion fracture of the distal phalanx

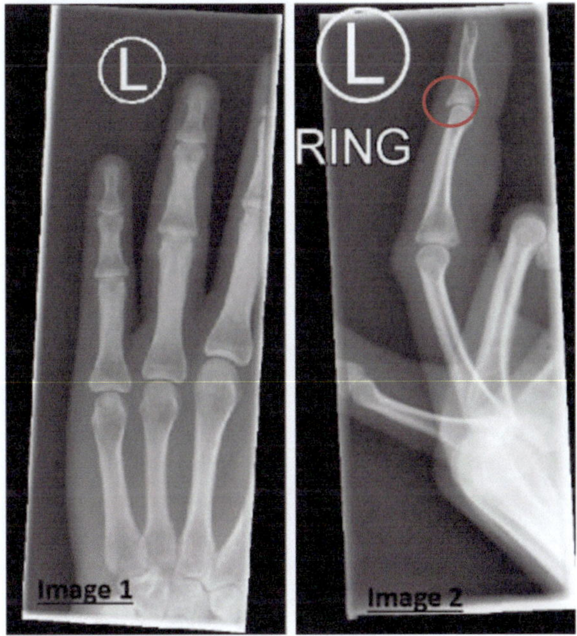

As seen in the DP view (image 1, shown in Fig. 1.3), the fracture is not fully visualised. However, in the lateral view (image 2, shown in Fig. 1.3), the fracture is clearly visible. This highlights the importance of using multiple projections and ensuring correct positioning.

1.3.3 Collateral Ligament Avulsion Fracture

An Avulsion Fracture located at the base of the middle phalanx can appear on either the medial or lateral aspect.

If the fracture is on the medial side, as seen in Fig. 1.4, it is described as an Ulnar Collateral Ligament Avulsion Fracture. If it is on the Lateral aspect, it is referred to as a Radial Collateral Ligament Avulsion Fracture [2].

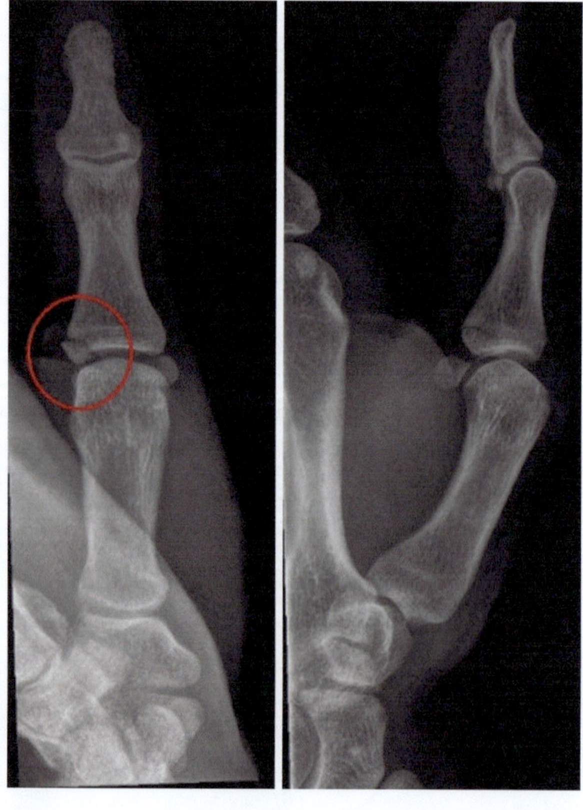

Fig. 1.4 Collateral ligament avulsion fracture at the base of the middle phalanx

1.3.4 Finger Dislocation

Finger dislocation occurs when the bones in a finger joint are displaced from their normal alignment. It usually occurs at the proximal interphalangeal (PIP) joint, which is demonstrated in Fig. 1.5 or the metacarpophalangeal (MCP) joint.

1.3.5 Seymour Fracture (AKA Tuft Injury)

Seymour fracture, also known as a tuft injury, is a distal phalanx physeal fracture often accompanied by a nail bed injury; this is illustrated in Fig. 1.6. It is a common finding in paediatric patients, usually resulting from crush injuries such as fingers caught in doors.

1.3.6 Games Keepers Thumb

This injury is typically caused by abduction and hyperextension of the thumb, leading to a rupture of the ulnar collateral ligament. An associated avulsion fracture may be visible at the lateral aspect of the base of the proximal phalanx.

This type of injury can result in difficulty or inability to perform a pinching motion, which is a key clinical sign.

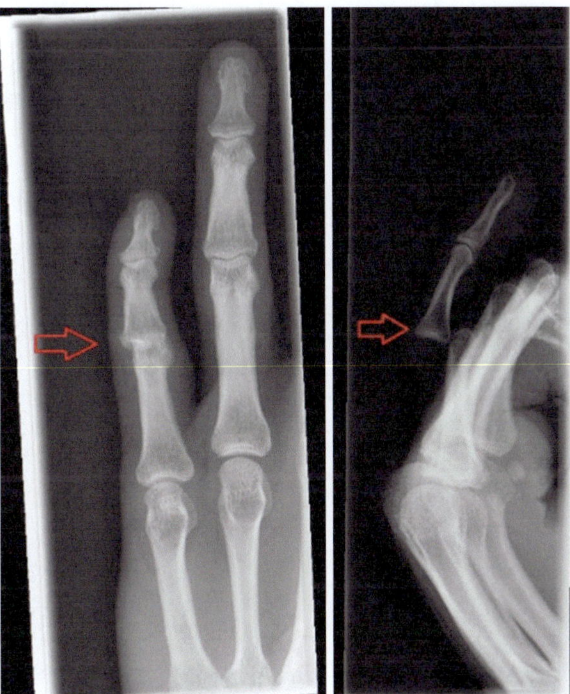

Fig. 1.5 Finger dislocation at the proximal interphalangeal joint

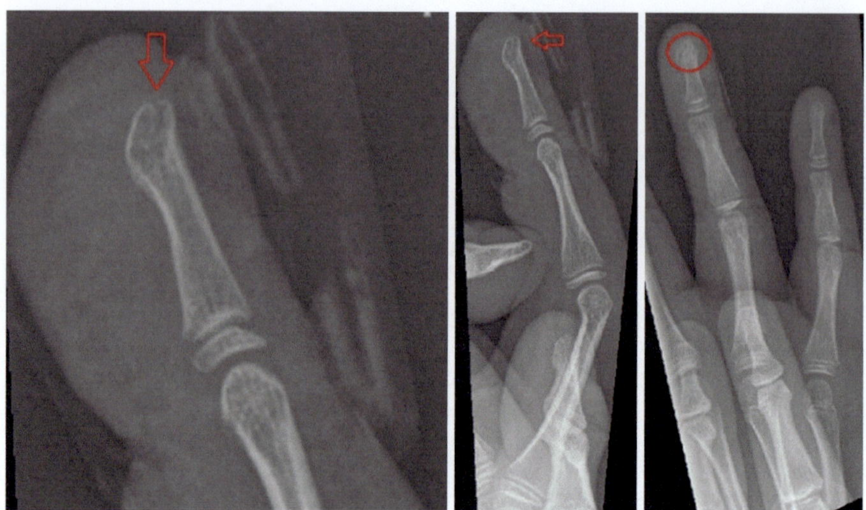

Fig. 1.6 Seymour Fracture of the distal phalanx

1.3.7 Mallet Finger

This is when the finger is stuck in flexion at the interphalangeal joint [3], most commonly at the distal interphalangeal joint. This injury is often associated with an extensor tendon avulsion fracture, as described above.

> Ligament injuries are often not associated with a fracture and may not always be visible on plain film imaging.

References

1. Whitley AS, Jefferson G, Holmes K, Sloane C, Anderson C. Clark's positioning in radiography. 13th ed. CRC Press; 2015.
2. Eiff MP, Hatch RL. Fracture management for primary care. 3rd ed. Saunders; 2012.
3. Greenspan A. Orthopedic imaging: A practical approach. 6th ed. Wolters Kluwer; 2015.

Hand

2

Figure 2.1 demonstrates the basic anatomical structures visible on both standard Dorsi-Palmar (DP) and Oblique Hand x-rays.

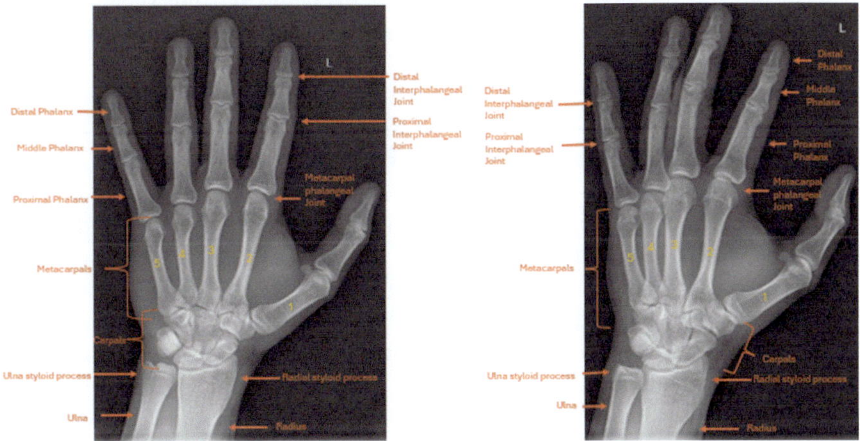

Fig. 2.1 Anatomical structures of the hand on the DP and Oblique views

2.1 Standard Views, Centring Points and Area of Interest

Dorsi Palmar The palmar aspect of the hand should be placed on the image receptor, with the fingers fully extended. The radial and ulnar styloid processes are equidistant, ensuring no rotation. The centring point is over the head of the third metacarpal.

Lateral Start with the palmar aspect of the hand placed flat on the image receptor, then externally rotate the hand 90 degrees to obtain a lateral view. The fingers should be completely extended, and the radial and ulnar styloid processes should be superimposed. The centring point is over the head of the second metacarpal.

Oblique Start with the palmar aspect of the hand placed flat on the image receptor, then externally rotate the hand 45 degrees to obtain an oblique view. The fingers will become slightly flexed and separated. The centring point is over the head of the second metacarpal.

Area of Interest In all views, the distal third of the radius and ulna should be visualised, extending distally to the fingertips. The lateral soft tissue borders must also be seen [3].

2.2 General Evaluation of Hand Examinations

1. The entire hand, including all phalanges, metacarpals, and the distal radius and ulna, should be included in the image.
2. The long axis of the hand should be aligned with the long axis of the image receptor to avoid distortion.
3. The image should be well-collimated to include the area of interest while minimising patient dose.
4. The positioning should demonstrate the standard views required (usually PA, oblique and lateral) with no overlapping of bones unless intended (e.g. oblique view).
5. The joint spaces (DIP, PIP, MCP and carpometacarpal joints) should be visible and open, indicating correct positioning.
6. The bony cortex and trabecular patterns should be sharp and well-defined, demonstrating adequate exposure and minimal motion blur.
7. Soft tissues should be visible enough to assess for swelling or foreign bodies.
8. There should be no motion or positioning artefacts obscuring the anatomy.
9. Evaluate for any pathology such as fractures, dislocations, degenerative changes or foreign bodies.

2.3   Common Hand Fractures/Pathologies

2.3.1   Bennetts Fracture

This fracture is demonstrated in Fig. 2.2. It is a fracture seen at the base of the first metacarpal that extends into the carpometacarpal joint, making it an intra-articular fracture.

This injury is usually caused by an axial force that is spread through a partially flexed thumb, commonly seen in falls or contact sports [2].

2.3.2   Reverse Bennett's Fracture

This is a fracture seen at the base of the fifth metacarpal that extends into the carpometacarpal joint, making it an intra-articular fracture. Figure 2.3 clearly demonstrates this fracture.

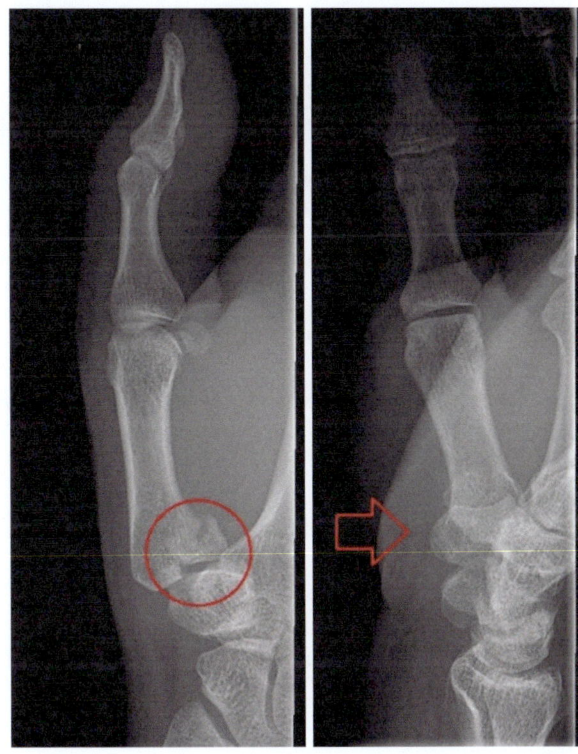

Fig. 2.2 Bennett's fracture at the base of the first metacarpal

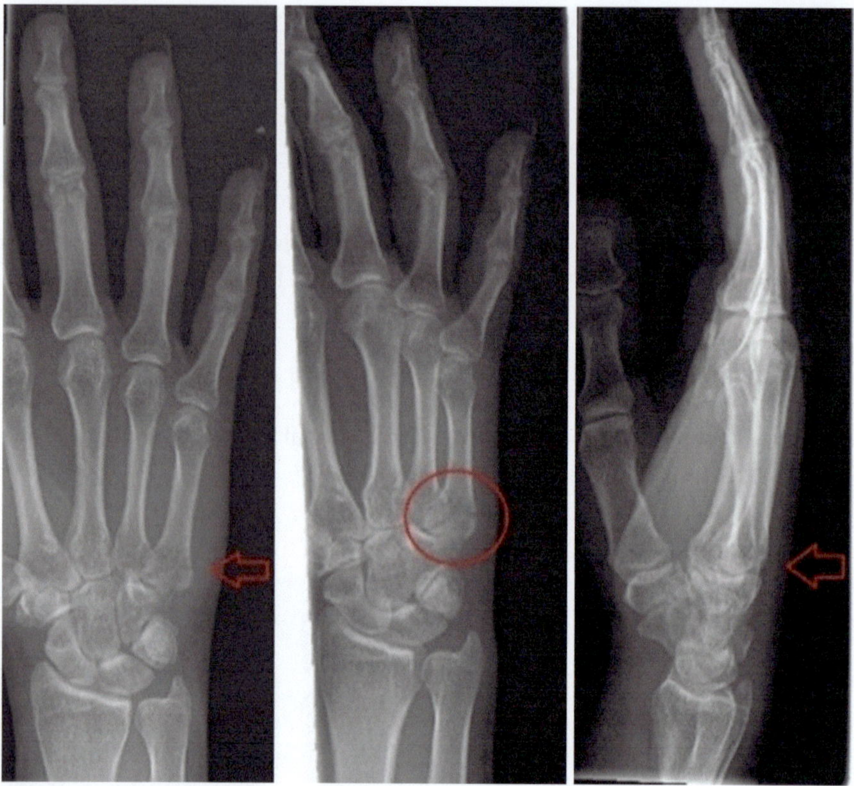

Fig. 2.3 Reverse Bennett's fracture at the base of the 5th metacarpal

2.3.3   Pseudo-Bennett Fracture

This is a fracture seen above the base of the first metacarpal; it does not extend into the carpometacarpal joint, making it an extra-articular fracture, shown in Fig. 2.4.

2.3.4   Rolando's Fracture

This is a fracture seen at the base of the first metacarpal that extends into the carpometacarpal joint, making it an intra-articular fracture. It is similar to a Bennett's Fracture, but in this case, it is a comminuted fracture, meaning that there are multiple fracture fragments.

   This injury is usually a result of high-impact trauma to the thumb and is demonstrated in Fig. 2.5.

Fig. 2.4 Pseudo-Bennett fracture above the base of the first metacarpal.

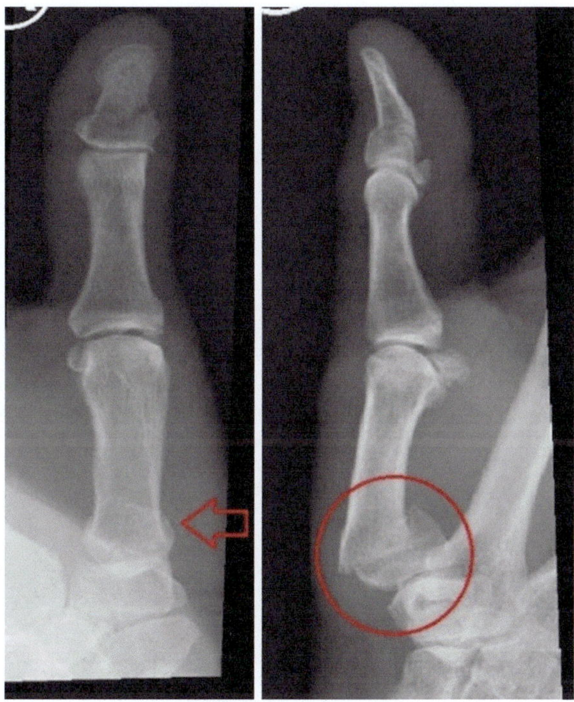

2.3.5   Boxers Fracture

This is a fracture, which, shown in Fig. 2.6, is typically seen at the neck of the fifth metacarpal, often accompanied by anterior angulation and may involve shortening of the metacarpal [1].

This injury typically results from a direct impact with a clenched fist, commonly referred to as a punch injury.

The fracture can be seen in the DP view; however, the fracture is more clearly visualised on the oblique view, where it appears anteriorly displaced (with the fracture fragment moved towards the palmar aspect of the hand). In the lateral view, you can see the sharp step in the cortex, indicating a break in the bone.

2.3.6   Metacarpal Fracture

Metacarpal fractures (Fig. 2.7) involve a break in one or more of the five metacarpal bones in the hand. Fractures in these bones can occur at the base, shaft, neck or head; they can also extend to the joints (intra-articular) or not extend to the joint (extra-articular).

Fig. 2.5 Rolando fracture at the base of the first metacarpal

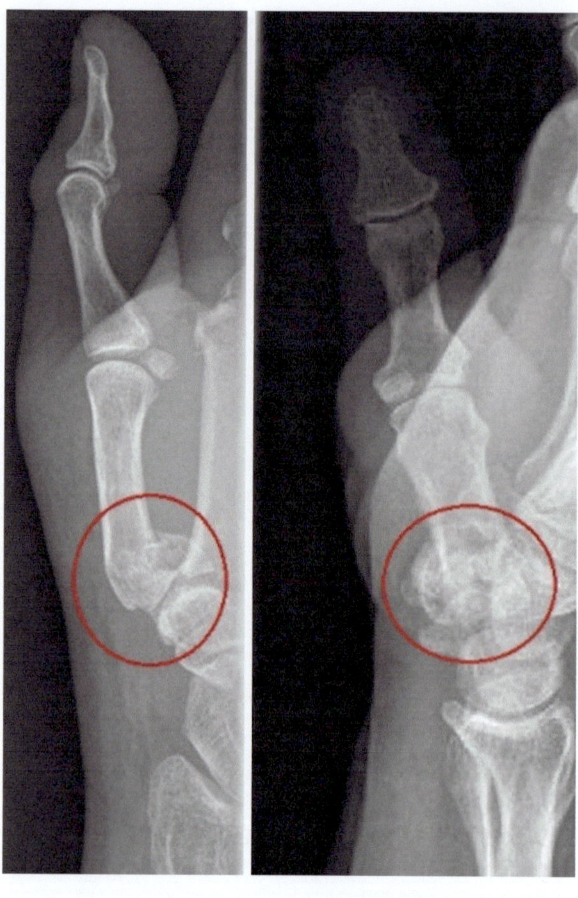

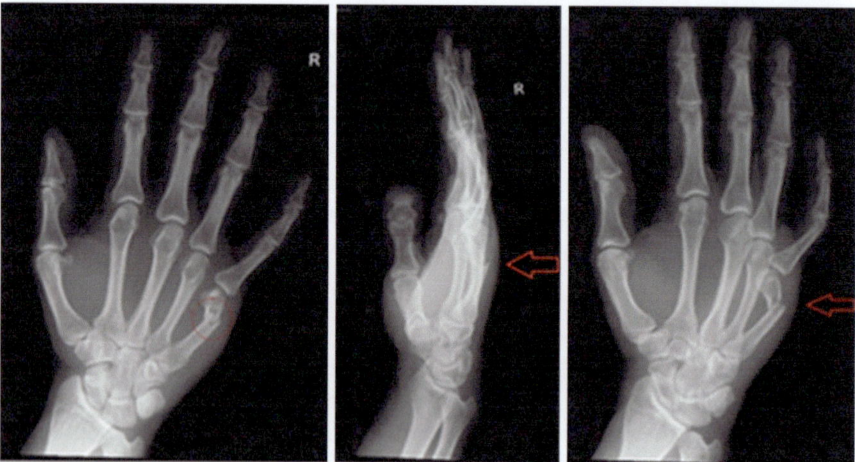

Fig. 2.6 Boxer's fracture of the fifth metacarpal neck

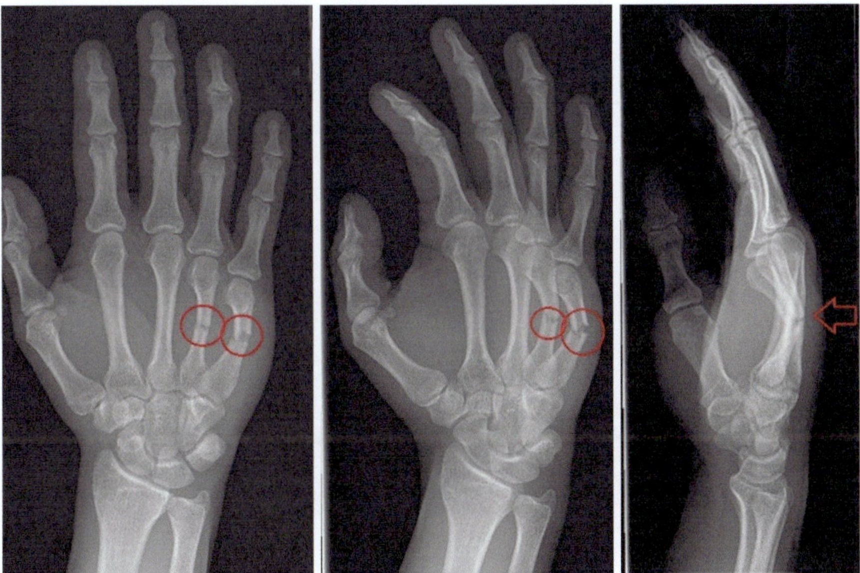

Fig. 2.7   Metacarpal Fractures seen at 4th and 5th MC

2.3.7   Carpo-Metacarpal (CMC) Dislocation

This is when there is a displacement of one or more of the metacarpal bases from the carpal bones at the carpometacarpal joint.

This injury is often caused by high-energy trauma such as road traffic accidents, falls or crush injuries.

Carpometacarpal dislocations usually occur at the fourth and fifth metacarpals, and some can be associated with fractures—these are referred to as fracture-dislocations.

Figure 2.8 uses all three hand projections—DP, Oblique and Lateral—to demonstrate this injury.

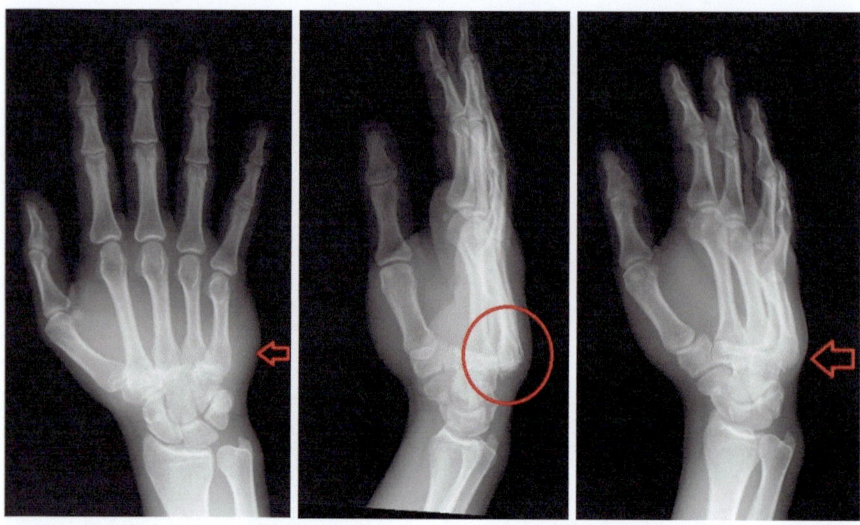

Fig. 2.8 CMC dislocation

References

1. Eiff MP, Hatch RL. Fracture management for primary care. 3rd ed. Saunders; 2012.
2. Greenspan A. Orthopedic imaging: a practical approach. 6th ed. Wolters Kluwer; 2015.
3. Whitley AS, Jefferson G, Holmes K, Sloane C, Anderson C. Clark's positioning in radiography. 13th ed. CRC Press; 2015.

Figure 3.1 demonstrates the basic anatomical structures visible on both standard Posteri-Anterior (PA) and Lateral wrist x-rays.

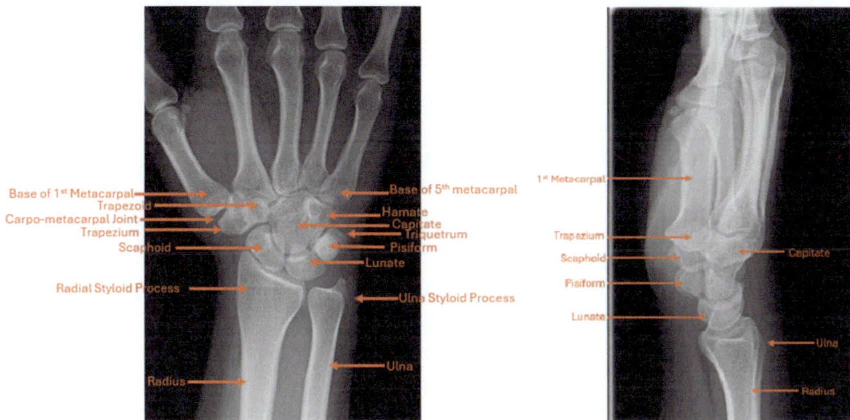

Fig. 3.1 Anatomical structures of the wrist on the PA and Lateral views

3.1   Standard Views, Centring Points and Area of Interest

Posteroanterior The anterior aspect of the forearm and the palmar aspect of the hand should be placed on the image receptor. The radial and ulnar styloid processes should be equidistant from the receptor to prevent rotation. The elbow joint can be flexed for comfort, with the shoulder, elbow and wrist in the same plane. The centring point should be midway between the radial and ulnar styloid processes.

Lateral From the Posteroanterior (PA) position, rotate the arm 90 degrees externally to achieve a lateral view. The elbow joint can be extended, and the shoulder, elbow, and wrist should be in the same plane. The radial and ulnar styloid processes should be superimposed to produce a true lateral.

> If the patient is in too much pain to achieve this position, lowering the table can help them externally rotate their hand to achieve a lateral position.

Area of Interest In both views, the distal third of the radius and ulna to the head of the metacarpals should be seen [3].

3.2   General Evaluation of Wrist Examinations

1. The entire wrist, including the distal radius, ulna, and all carpal bones, should be fully visible and properly centred on the image receptor.
2. The wrist should be positioned straight with appropriate collimation focused on the area of interest to minimise patient dose.
3. Standard views (PA, lateral and oblique) should be taken to ensure comprehensive visualisation of all wrist structures.
4. Joint spaces between the carpal bones, radius and ulna should be open, uniform and visible.
5. The carpal bones should appear in two distinct rows, held in place by surrounding ligaments.
6. On the PA view, the three carpal arcs—formed by the proximal and distal carpal rows—should show smooth, continuous curves without any disruption.
7. The intercarpal joint spaces should be uniform, typically measuring 1–2 mm. Any increase suggests possible displacement from ligament disruption, which may be evident on the PA projection.
8. On the lateral view, a straight line should pass through the bases of the metacarpal, Capitate, Lunate and distal radius.
9. Any disruption of this alignment suggests dislocation, and it is important to note which bone is displaced or misaligned.
10. The bone edges and trabecular patterns should be sharp and clear, with no blurring or motion artefacts.

11. Soft tissues should be visible enough to assess for swelling or other abnormalities.
12. The image should be free from artefacts or technical issues that could obscure important details.
13. Carefully evaluate for fractures, dislocations, ligament injuries or other pathologies.

3.3 Common Wrist Fractures/Pathologies

3.3.1 Lunate Dislocation

Lunate dislocation is illustrated in Fig. 3.2, where the lunate is displaced anteriorly (volar) and no longer articulates with the distal radius [2]. The capitate sits posterior to the lunate, distinguishing this injury from a perilunate dislocation (described on page 27, shown in Fig. 3.3).

This dislocation is considered severe as it typically involves all of the intercarpal joints and can disrupt most of the major carpal ligaments. It can also be associated with a scaphoid fracture.

Widening of the Scaphoid-Lunate intercarpal joint would be suggestive of a ligament injury.

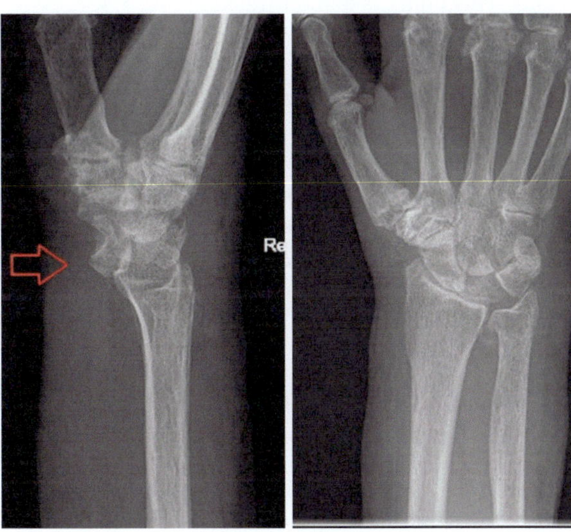

Fig. 3.2 Lunate dislocation

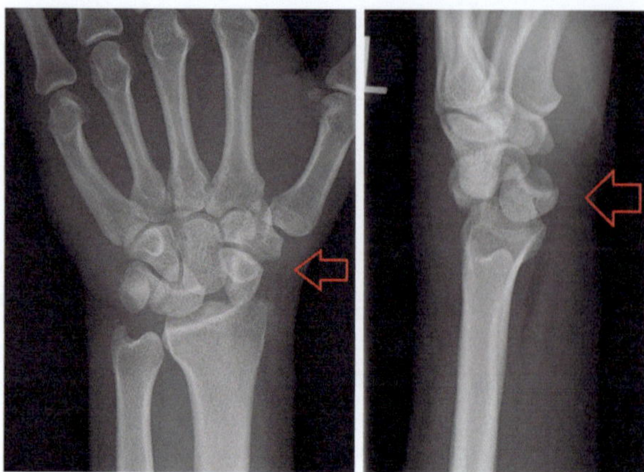

Fig. 3.3 Perilunate dislocation

3.3.2   Perilunate Dislocation

The capitate and adjacent carpal bones are posteriorly displaced from the lunate, while the lunate remains in line with the distal radius.

This injury is demonstrated in Fig. 3.3.

> This injury may also be linked to a scaphoid fracture; it is equally important to assess for fractures of the ulnar styloid process.

3.3.3   Midcarpal Dislocation

The lunate and capitate both become displaced. The capitate is dislocated from the lunate, and the lunate shows a partial dislocation (subluxation) from the distal radius. This injury is demonstrated in Fig. 3.4.

3.3.4   Dorsal Triquetral Fracture

An avulsion fracture is seen at the dorsal aspect of the triquetrum, visualised in Fig. 3.5. This is the most commonly seen triquetral fracture.

This fracture is often described as the pooping duck sign, as the triquetrum resembles the body of a duck, and the avulsion fracture resembles a small droplet behind it. This helps recognise the injury as it can be easily missed on a plain film image.

> Note that triquetral fractures can also occur at the body of the triquetrum as well as the volar aspect of the triquetrum. While these injuries are less common, it is still essential to be aware of them.

Fig. 3.4 Midcarpal dislocation

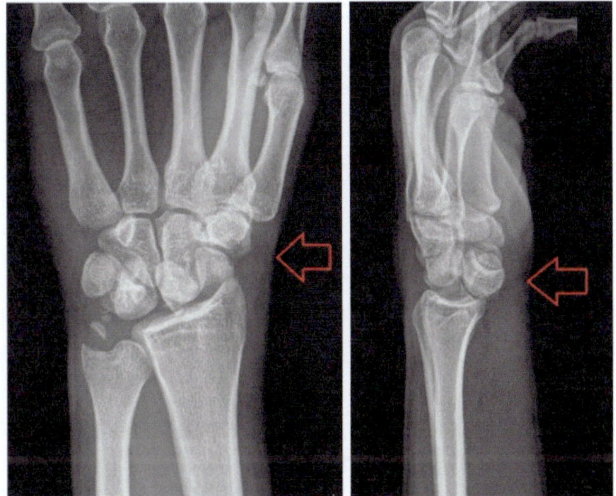

Fig. 3.5 Dorsal triquetral fracture

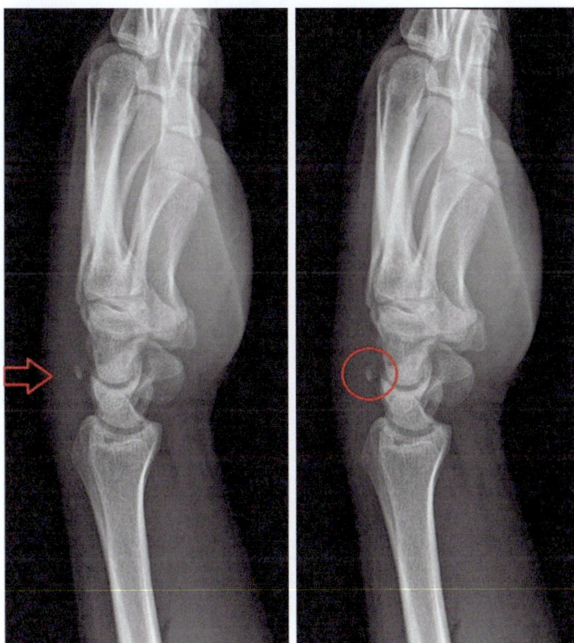

3.3.5 Chauffeur's Fracture

This is a fracture involving the Radial Styloid process, which extends to the radio-carpal joint space, making it an intra-articular fracture (Fig. 3.6). The fracture fragment is mildly displaced, and no changes are seen in the carpal bones/joints [1].

Fig. 3.6 Chauffeur's
fracture

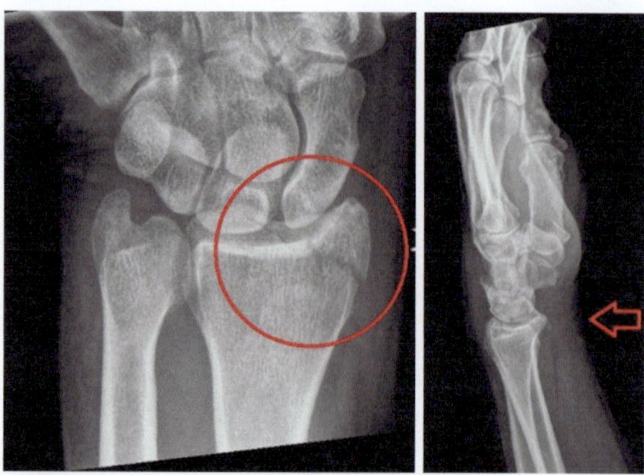

Fig. 3.7 Colles fracture

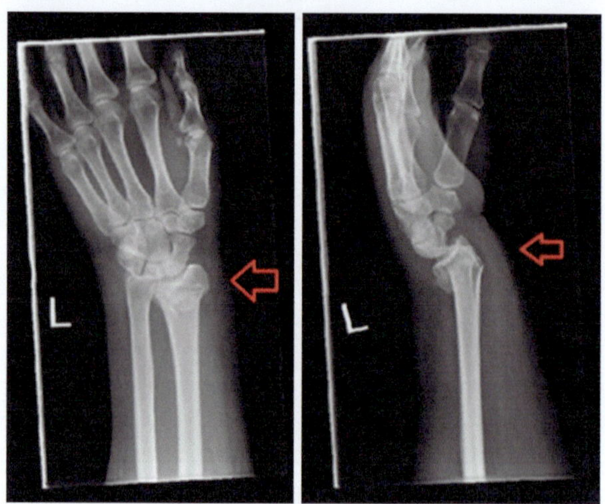

3.3.6   Colles Fracture

This is an extra-articular transverse fracture of the distal radius and ulna. The distal
fracture fragments are displaced and angulated posteriorly, as demonstrated in
Fig. 3.7. This pattern typically results from a fall onto an outstretched hand
(FOOSH).

3.3.7   Smith's Fracture

This is an extra-articular transverse fracture of the distal radius and ulna. The distal
fracture fragments are displaced and angulated anteriorly, as demonstrated in
Fig. 3.8. This type of injury typically results from a fall onto a flexed wrist or a
direct blow to the dorsal aspect of the wrist.

Fig. 3.8 Smith's fracture

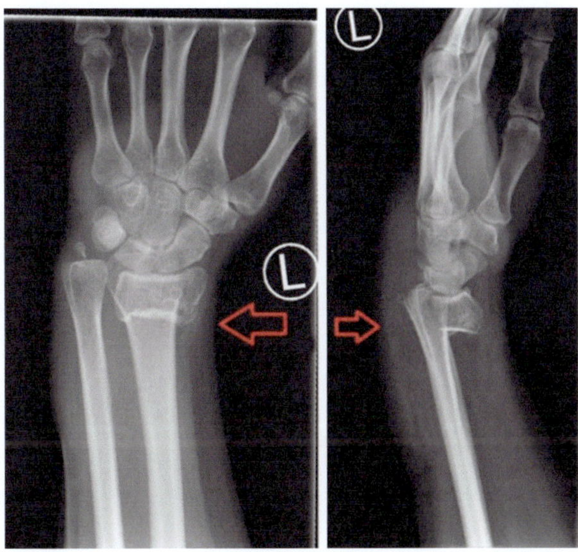

References

1. Eiff MP, Hatch RL. Fracture management for primary care. 3rd ed. Saunders; 2012.
2. Greenspan A. Orthopedic imaging: a practical approach. 6th ed. Wolters Kluwer; 2015.
3. Whitley AS, Jefferson G, Holmes K, Sloane C, Anderson C. Clark's positioning in radiography. 13th ed. CRC Press; 2015.

Scaphoid

4

Figure 4.1 demonstrates the basic anatomical structures of the scaphoid visible on an X-ray.

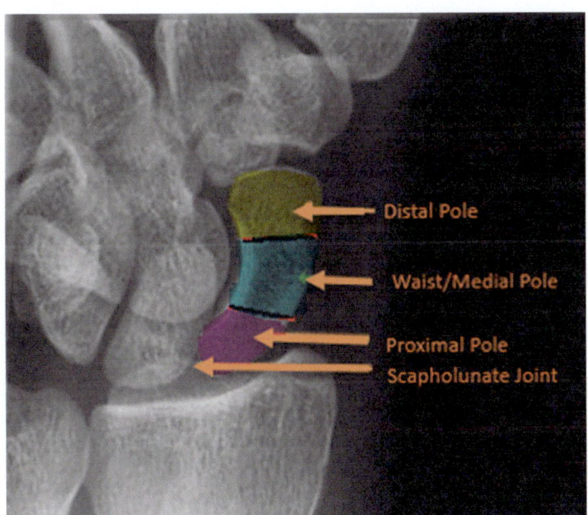

Fig. 4.1 Anatomical structures of the scaphoid

S. Moughal, *Fracture Finder: A Practical Guide to Interpreting Upper and Lower Limb X-Rays for Radiographers*,
https://doi.org/10.1007/978-3-032-17324-9_4

4.1   Standard Views, Centring Points and Area of Interest

Postero-anterior The anterior aspect of the forearm and the palmar aspect of the hand should be placed on the image receptor. The radial and ulnar styloid processes should be equidistant from the receptor to prevent rotation. The elbow joint can be flexed for comfort, with the shoulder, elbow and wrist in the same plane. The centring point should be midway between the radial and ulnar styloid processes.

Posterior-Anterior with Ulnar Deviation Position the wrist as for the standard PA view, then deviate the wrist towards the ulnar. This elongates the scaphoid and brings it out of superimposition. The centring point should be midway between the radius and ulnar styloid processes.

Posterior-Anterior with Ulnar Deviation with Tube Angulation As with the PA ulnar deviation view, position the wrist with ulnar deviation. Then, angle the x-ray tube 15–20° cranially and centre over the scaphoid. This further elongates the scaphoid to enhance the visualisation of the scaphoid waist.

Oblique Start in the PA position, then externally rotate the wrist 45 degrees to obtain an oblique view. This view offers an additional angle for evaluating the scaphoid and its surrounding carpal bones.

Lateral From the (PA) position, rotate the arm 90 degrees externally to achieve a lateral view. The elbow joint can be extended, and the shoulder, elbow and wrist should be in the same plane. The radial and ulnar styloid processes should be superimposed to produce a true lateral. The centring point should be on the radial styloid process [1].

Area of Interest For the PA, oblique and lateral views, the area of interest will be the distal third of the radius and ulna to the head of the metacarpals.

The PA with ulnar deviation and PA ulnar deviation with tube angulation; the area of interest is the scaphoid, so include the distal radius, ulna and the base of the metacarpals to focus more on the scaphoid while allowing the assessment of the carpal alignment.

4.2   General Evaluation of Scaphoid Examinations

1. The entire scaphoid bone should be visible, including its waist and both proximal and distal poles.
2. Images should include standard scaphoid views such as PA with ulnar deviation, lateral and oblique projections to best visualise the scaphoid.
3. The scaphoid should be well-centred on the image receptor, with appropriate collimation to focus on the wrist area and minimise patient dose.
4. Joint spaces around the scaphoid, especially the scapholunate interval, should be uniform and clearly defined. Any widening may suggest ligament injury.

5. The trabecular pattern and cortical outline of the scaphoid should be sharp and uninterrupted to detect subtle fractures.
6. On the lateral view, assess the alignment of the scaphoid with the other carpal bones; disruption may indicate dislocation or fracture displacement.
7. Soft tissue shadows should be evaluated for signs of swelling or trauma.
8. The image should be free of motion artefacts and technical faults that could obscure detail.
9. Evaluate for signs of scaphoid fractures, avascular necrosis or other pathology.

4.3 Common Scaphoid Fracture/Pathologies

4.3.1 Scaphoid Fracture

The most commonly seen scaphoid fracture is a transverse fracture seen through the waist of the scaphoid, shown in Fig. 4.2. Less common fractures are seen at the proximal, demonstrated in Fig. 4.3, and distal ends of the pole. The images below show both midshaft and proximal scaphoid fractures.

Fractures that occur closer to the proximal pole of the scaphoid have a poorer healing rate [2]. This is because it will leave the fracture fragment with no blood supply, as the scaphoid only has a blood supply from one direction.

Plain film imaging has a lower sensitivity in detecting scaphoid fractures. If the fracture is not visible on a plain film, but there is still suspicion, then a CT or MRI scan may be suggested.

Midshaft/Waist Scaphoid Fracture

Proximal Pole Scaphoid Fracture

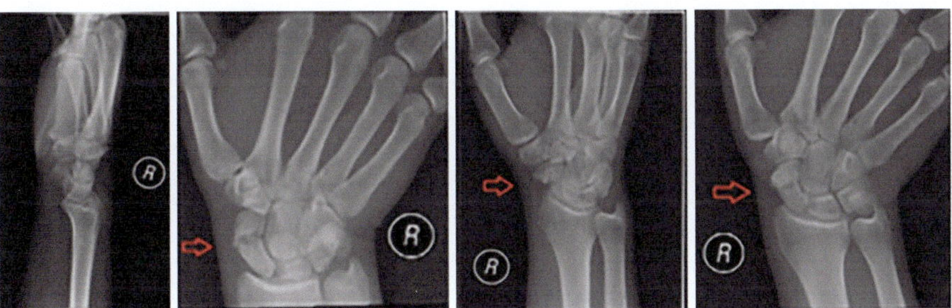

Fig. 4.2 Midshaft scaphoid fracture

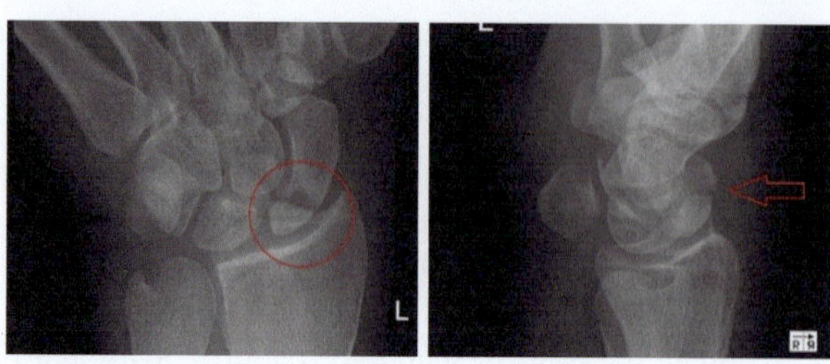

Fig. 4.3 Proximal pole scaphoid fracture

References

1. Bontrager KL, Lampignano JP. Textbook of radiographic positioning and related anatomy. 9th ed. Elsevier; 2018.
2. Greenspan A. Orthopedic imaging: a practical approach. 6th ed. Wolters Kluwer; 2015.

Forearm

5

Figure 5.1 demonstrates the basic anatomical structures visible on both standard antero-posterior (AP) and lateral forearm x-rays.

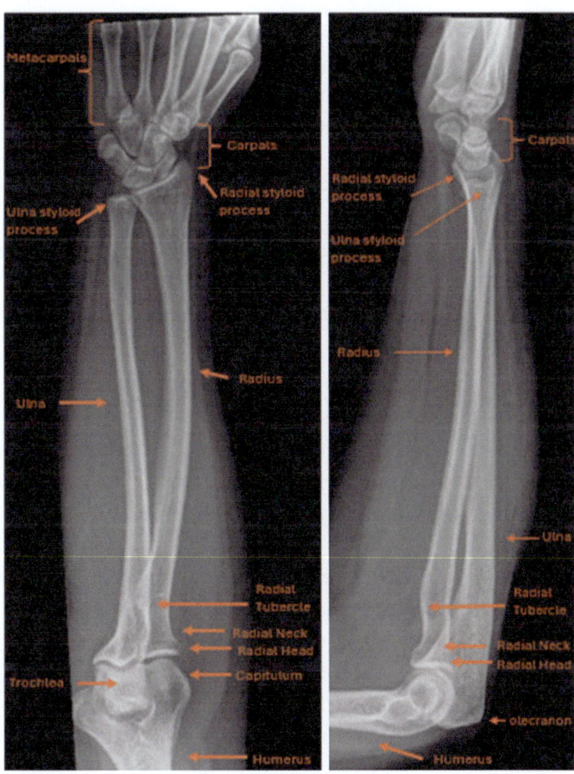

Fig. 5.1 Anatomical structures of the forearm on the AP and lateral views

S. Moughal, *Fracture Finder: A Practical Guide to Interpreting Upper and Lower Limb X-Rays for Radiographers*,
https://doi.org/10.1007/978-3-032-17324-9_5

5.1   Standard Views, Centring Points and Area of Interest

Antero-posterior The forearm should be supinated, resting on the image receptor. The arm should be abducted with the elbow joint fully extended. The styloid processes should be equidistant. The centring point is midway between the elbow and wrist joint.

Lateral From the anteroposterior position, the elbow should be flexed at 90° with the ulnar aspect of the forearm resting on the image receptor. The humerus is rotated to bring the medial aspect of the upper arm, the elbow, the forearm, the wrist and the hand in contact with the image receptor. The radial and ulnar styloid processes should be superimposed. The centring point is midway between the elbow and wrist joint.

Area of Interest In both views, the radius and ulna should be seen completely, including the whole aspect of the wrist and elbow joint. The lateral soft tissue borders should also be included [1].

5.2   General Evaluation of Forearm Examinations

1. The entire forearm should be visible on the image, including the wrist joint distally and the elbow joint proximally.
2. The forearm should be positioned so that the long axis of the radius and ulna is aligned with the image receptor to avoid distortion.
3. Appropriate collimation should be used to include the entire forearm and minimise patient dose.
4. Standard views typically include AP (anteroposterior) and lateral projections to assess both bones.
5. The cortical outlines and trabecular patterns of the radius and ulna should be sharp, with no motion blur.
6. Wrist and elbow joints should be visible and free from overlapping structures.
7. Assess soft tissues for swelling, foreign bodies, or other abnormalities.
8. Look carefully for fractures, dislocations, or any deformities of the bones or joints.
9. The image should be free of artefacts or positioning errors that may obscure critical anatomy.

The radius and ulna form a ring-like structure with the distal and proximal radioulnar joints. Due to this structure, a fracture in one part of the ring often indicates another elsewhere in the structure. This is why it is important to assess the entire forearm, including both joints, for additional injuries if a fracture is identified.

5.3   Common Forearm Fracture/Pathologies

5.3.1   Impacted Radius

This is an impacted distal radius fracture. There is trabecular crowding and overlapping of fracture ends, which is consistent with impaction. There will be a slight increase in bone density, indicated by a sclerotic line, as demonstrated Fig. 5.2.

5.3.2   Barton Fracture

This is an intra-articular fracture of the rim of the distal radius, which has an associated dislocation or subluxation of the radiocarpal joint. This feature distinguishes it from a Colles' or Smith's fracture, which are typically extra-articular without joint dislocation. This injury is demonstrated in Fig. 5.3.

5.3.3   Torus Fracture (AKA a Buckle Fracture)

A torus fracture is an incomplete fracture; it occurs when one side of the bone buckles or compresses without breaking it completely. It is primarily seen in children. Figure 5.4 visualises this fracture clearly.

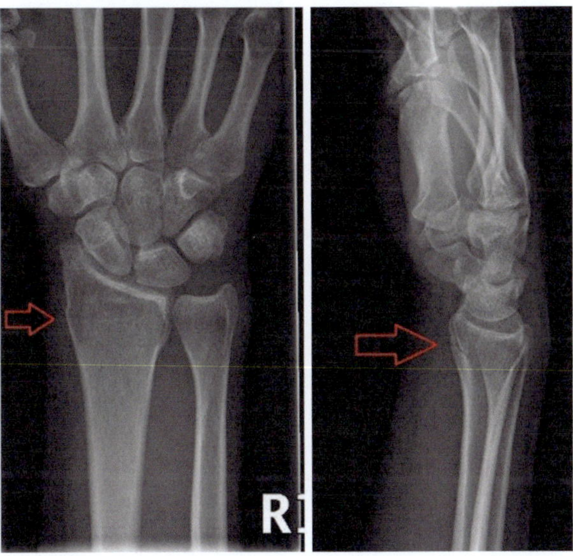

Fig. 5.2 Impacted radius fracture

Fig. 5.3 Barton fracture

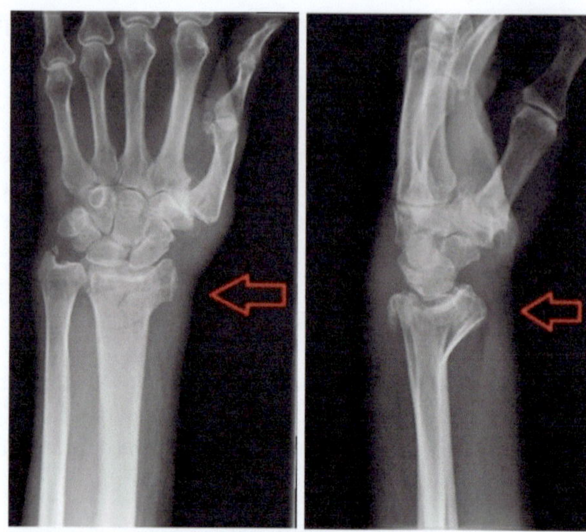

Fig. 5.4 Torus fracture

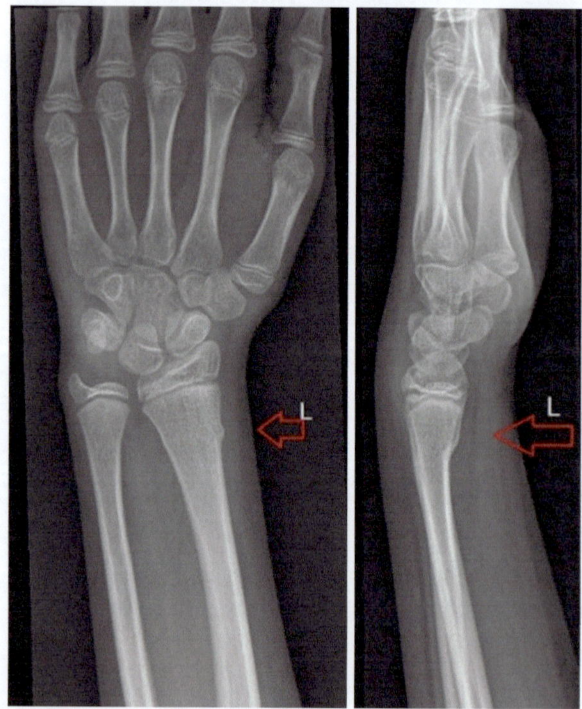

5.3.4 Monteggia Fracture

This is a fracture dislocation injury demonstrated in Fig. 5.5. This injury involves a fracture seen at the proximal or midshaft of the ulna with a dislocation of the radial head [2].

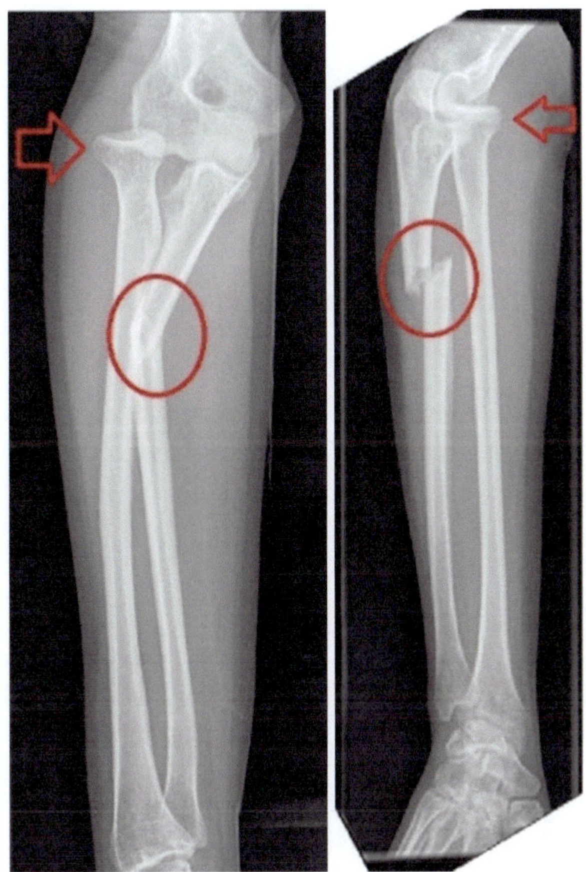

Fig. 5.5 Monteggia fracture

5.3.5   Galeazzi Fracture

There are various classifications of Monteggia fractures, which depend on the direction of the radial head dislocation and the type of ulnar fracture. The most widely accepted system is the Bado Classification, divided into four types.

This is a fracture-dislocation involving the distal or mid-shaft radius, accompanied by a dislocation of the distal radioulnar joint (Fig. 5.6).

The injury typically results from a fall onto an outstretched hand with the forearm in a pronated position.

Fig. 5.6 Galeazzi fracture

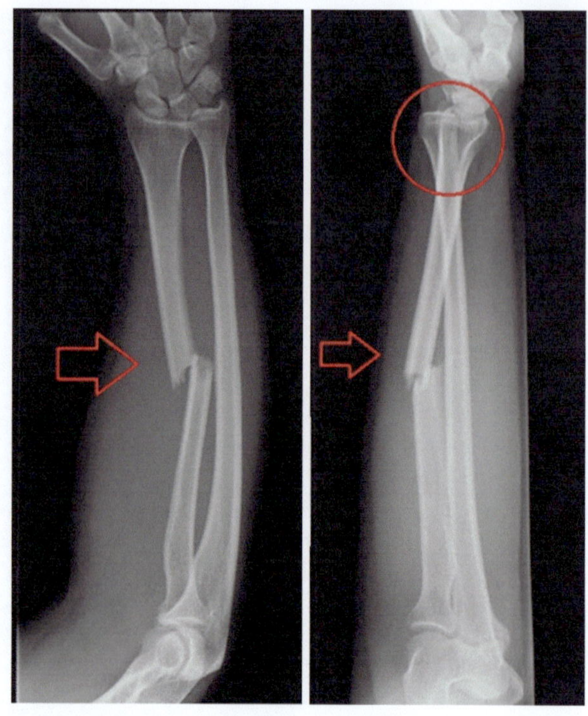

References

1. Whitley AS, Jefferson G, Holmes K, Sloane C, Anderson C. Clark's positioning in radiography. 13th ed. CRC Press; 2015.
2. Carver E, Carver B. Medical imaging: techniques, reflection & evaluation. 2nd ed. Wiley-Blackwell; 2012.

Elbow 6

Figure 6.1 demonstrates the basic anatomical structures visible on both standard antero-posterior (AP) and lateral elbow x-rays.

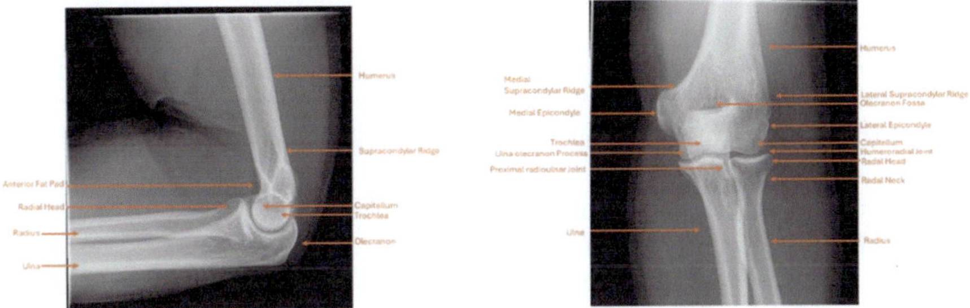

Fig. 6.1 Anatomical structures of the elbow on the AP and Lateral views

6.1   Standard Views, Centring Points and Area of Interest

Antero-posterior The forearm should be extended with the posterior aspect of the elbow in contact with the image receptor. The humeral epicondyles should be equidistant, with the shoulder, elbow and wrist in the same plane of motion.

The centring point is midway between the humeral epicondyles.

Lateral The forearm should be externally rotated and the elbow flexed 90°. The medial aspect of the elbow should be in contact with the image receptor. The shoulder, elbow and wrist should all be in the same plane. The medial and lateral epicondyles should be superimposed.

The centring point is over the lateral epicondyle.

Area of Interest In both views, the distal third of the humerus and the proximal third of the elbow should be visible.

6.2   General Evaluation of Elbow Examinations

1. The entire elbow joint should be visible, including the distal humerus, proximal radius and ulna.
2. Images should include the standard views: AP, lateral and often oblique projections to assess the joint fully.
3. Proper positioning and collimation are essential to ensure the elbow is centred and well visualised while minimising patient dose.
4. Bone edges and trabecular patterns should be sharp and clear, with no motion blur or artefacts.
5. Soft tissues should be examined for signs of swelling or injury.

Specific to Assessing Elbow Images
When evaluating elbow images, it is crucial to look for subtle signs that could indicate an occult (hidden) fracture. Examining fat pads and alignment lines is crucial [1].

Fat Pad Signs (Shown in Fig. 6.2)
1. *Anterior fat pad*—this is usually visible on a lateral elbow X-ray. However, if it is elevated or sail-shaped (known as the sail sign), this suggests a joint effusion, which is typically caused by an occult fracture.
2. *Posterior Fat Pad*—This is not ordinarily visible. When it is seen, it usually indicates a joint effusion, which occurs due to intra-articular fractures.
3. This is demonstrated in Fig. 6.2

Fig. 6.2 Visualisation of
fat pad and sail sign

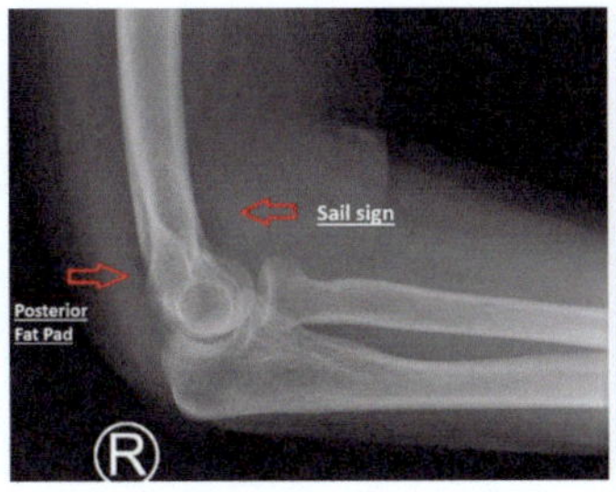

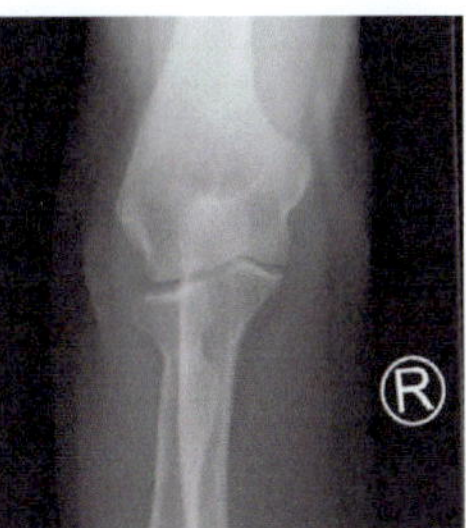

Alignment Checks
4. *Anterior Humeral Line*—on the lateral projection, a line should run along
   the anterior surface of the humeral shaft. It should meet the middle third of
   the capitellum. If it does not, then an injury should be considered (commonly a supracondylar fracture)
5. *Capitellar Line*—In both AP and lateral projections, a line should run
   through the centre of the radial neck and shaft and pass through the centre
   of the capitellum. Misalignment would suggest a fracture or dislocation
   (commonly a radial head injury).

6.3   Common Elbow Fracture/Pathologies

6.3.1   Medial Epicondyle Fracture

This fracture, which is demonstrated in Fig. 6.3, usually involves an avulsion injury
of the medial epicondyle of the humerus and is commonly seen in paediatric
patients. The fracture fragment may be displaced superiorly and laterally, often
visualised overlying the capitellum.

6.3.2   Lateral Epicondyle Fracture

This fracture typically involves an avulsion injury of the lateral epicondyle of the
humerus and is less common than medial epicondyle fractures. The fracture fragment may appear displaced laterally and proximally. This type of injury is demonstrated in Fig. 6.4, as shown on a paediatric x-ray.

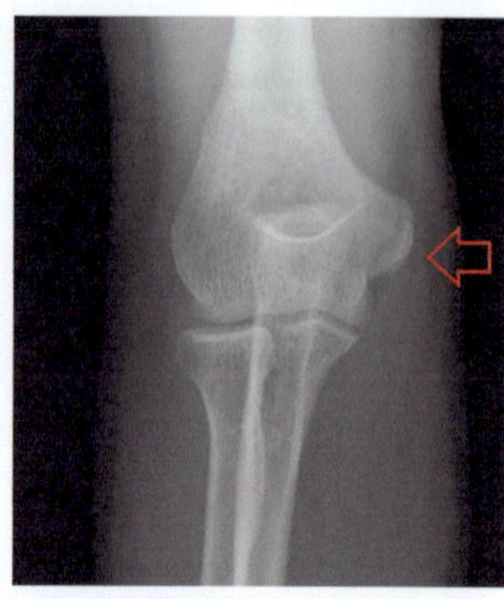

Fig. 6.3 Medial epicondyle fracture

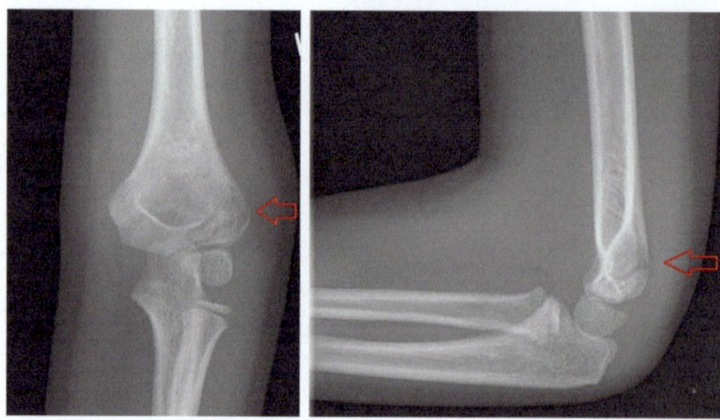

Fig. 6.4 Lateral epicondyle fracture

6.3.3   Radial Head Fracture

The image above shows the fracture on a paediatric elbow. When assessing paediatric elbow trauma, it is important to recognise the ossification centres to avoid mistaking them for fractures. These centres appear in a predictable order, remembered with the mnemonic CRITOL:

1. Capitellum—appears around 1 year
2. Radial head—appears around 3 years
3. Internal (medial) epicondyle—appears around 5 years
4. Trochlea—appears around 7 years
5. Olecranon—appears around 9 years
6. Lateral epicondyle—appears around 11 years

Fig. 6.5 Radial head fracture

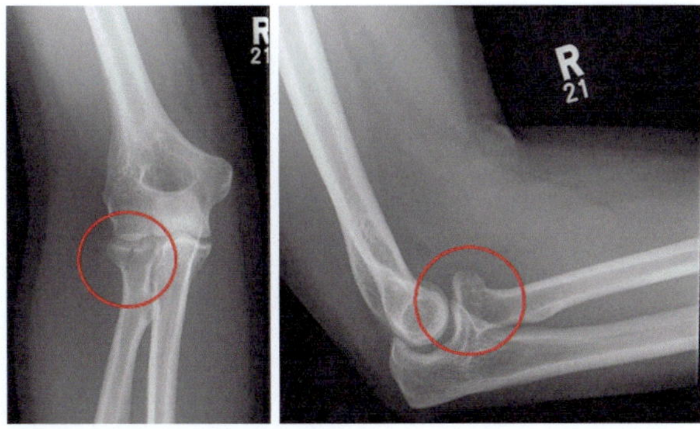

There are four common types of Radial Head Fracture, which are listed and described below. Figure 6.5 illustrates an example of a radial head fracture. An intra-articular oblique fracture is seen through the radial head with minimal anterior displacement of the fracture fragment, classifying it as a shear radial head fracture.

6.3.4   Supracondylar Fracture

There are four common types of radial head fractures:

Split Fracture—This is a linear fracture through the radial head mostly seen without displacement.
Shear Fracture—this is often an oblique fracture through the radial head often seen with anterior displacement of the fracture fragment.
Tilted or Angulated Fracture—This is when the radial head is tilted or angulating causing it to affect the joint alignment. There is usually no fracture fragment.
Crush Fracture—this is a comminuted fracture of the radial head—multiple fracture fragments seen.

There is a transverse fracture through the distal humeral metaphysis (just proximal to the epicondyles)—this is consistent with a supracondylar fracture. The distal fracture fragment appears posteriorly displaced. This is demonstrated in Fig. 6.6.

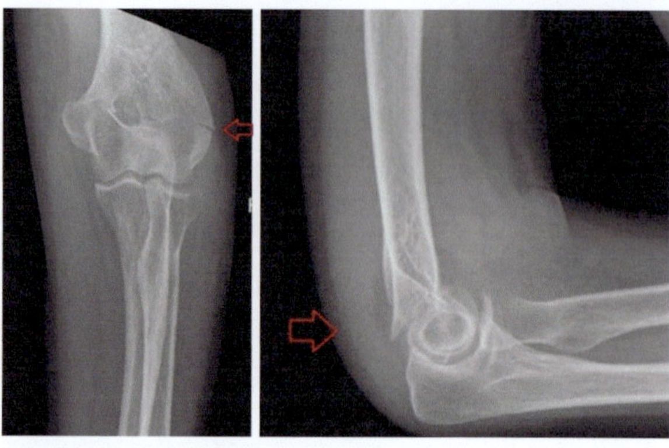

Fig. 6.6 Supracondylar fracture

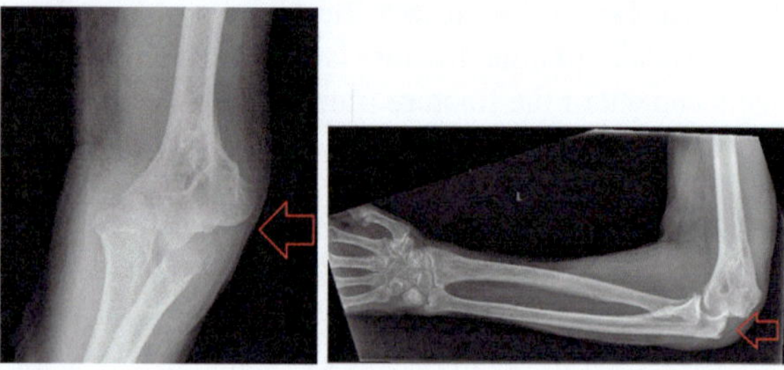

Fig. 6.7 Anterior elbow dislocation

6.3.5 Anterior Elbow Dislocation

Depending on the type of injury, the fracture fragment can be posteriorly or anteriorly displaced:

An extension-type injury would cause posterior displacement
A flexion-type injury would cause anterior displacement.

There is an anterior displacement of the radius and ulna corresponding to the distal aspect of the humerus (Fig. 6.7). The radius and ulna are seen anterior to the humerus.

6.3.6 Posterior Elbow Dislocation

There is a posterior displacement of the radius and ulna corresponding to the distal aspect of the humerus (Fig. 6.8). The radius and ulna are seen posterior to the humerus.

Fig. 6.8 Posterior elbow dislocation

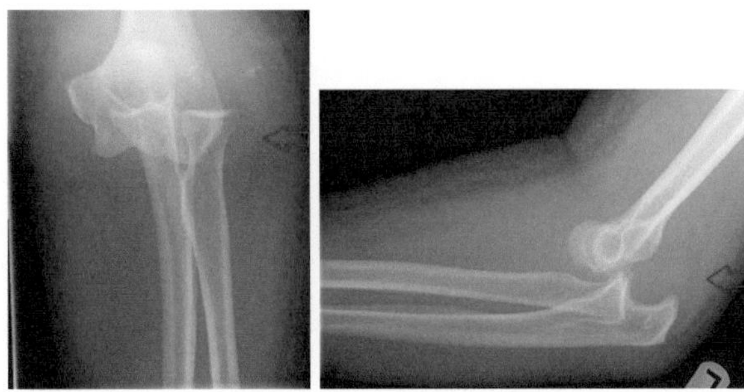

Reference

1. Greenspan A. Orthopedic imaging: a practical approach. 6th ed. Wolters Kluwer; 2015.

Humerus 7

7.1 Standard Views, Centring Points and Area of Interest

Antero-posterior The posterior aspect of the arm should be in contact with the image receptor. The arm should be fully extended with the hand in a supinated position, which opens the glenohumeral joint. Humeral epicondyles should be equidistant. The centring point is the midshaft of the humerus.

Lateral From the AP position, rotate the patient until the lateral aspect of the affected arm is in contact with the image receptor. The elbow should be flexed to 90°, with the hand placed on the hip, if the patient can tolerate this position. This ensures the epicondyles are perpendicular to the image receptor, providing an accurate lateral projection of the humerus.

The centring point is the midshaft of the humerus.

Area of Interest In both views, the humerus should be visualised completely, with the glenohumeral and elbow joint included.

7.2 General Evaluation of Humerus Examinations

1. The entire humerus must be included, from the shoulder joint (including the glenoid) to the elbow joint (including the olecranon and distal humerus).
2. The midshaft of the humerus should be demonstrated with no cut-off at either joint.
3. The bony cortex and trabecular pattern should be visible, indicating appropriate exposure and contrast.
4. Soft tissue structures should be visible to assess for swelling or displacement.

© The Author(s), under exclusive license to Springer Nature Switzerland AG 2026
S. Moughal, *Fracture Finder: A Practical Guide to Interpreting Upper and Lower Limb X-Rays for Radiographers*,
https://doi.org/10.1007/978-3-032-17324-9_7

7.3   Common Humerus Fracture/Pathologies

7.3.1   Greater Tuberosity Fracture

This is a fracture involving the greater tuberosity of the humerus. It can be displaced, with bony fragments often visualised lateral to the humeral head (as seen in Fig. 7.1). This type of fracture is commonly associated with anterior shoulder dislocations.

7.3.2   Surgical Neck Fracture

These fractures carry a high risk of rotator cuff injury, particularly involving the supraspinatus tendon.

This fracture is commonly seen as a transverse or oblique break with angulation and displacement through the surgical neck, just below the greater and lesser tuberosities.

These fractures carry a high risk of axillary nerve injury, so it is important to assess for sensory loss over the deltoid region during clinical examination.

In the image below (Fig. 7.2), a transverse fracture is seen through the surgical neck of the humerus.

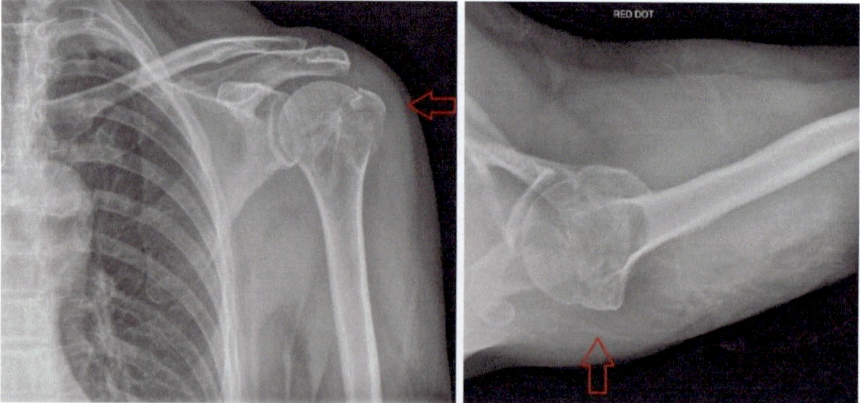

Fig. 7.1   Greater tuberosity fracture

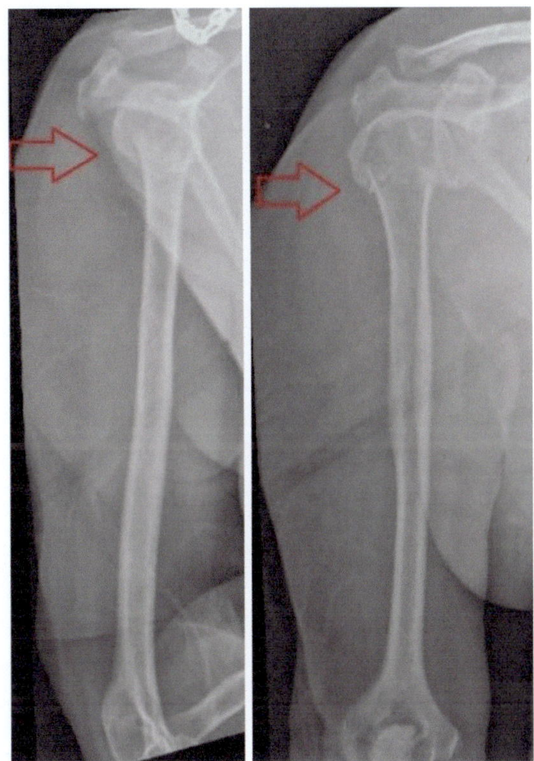

Fig. 7.2 Surgical neck fracture

7.3.3   Anatomical Neck Fracture

This is a fracture separating the humeral head from the greater and lesser tuberosities. The illustration below demonstrates the injury clearly (Fig. 7.3).

7.3.4   Midshaft Fracture

> These fractures carry a high risk of avascular necrosis as it causes disruption to the arcuate artery [1].

This is a fracture that occurs at the midshaft of the humerus. These fractures can appear transverse, spiral, oblique or comminuted.

Figure 7.4 demonstrates a spiral fracture seen at the distal aspect of the humeral shaft.

Fig. 7.3 Drawing of an anatomical neck fracture

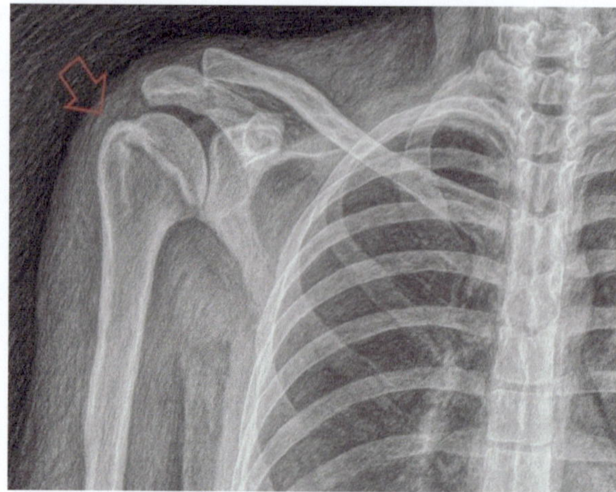

Fig. 7.4 Humeral midshaft fracture

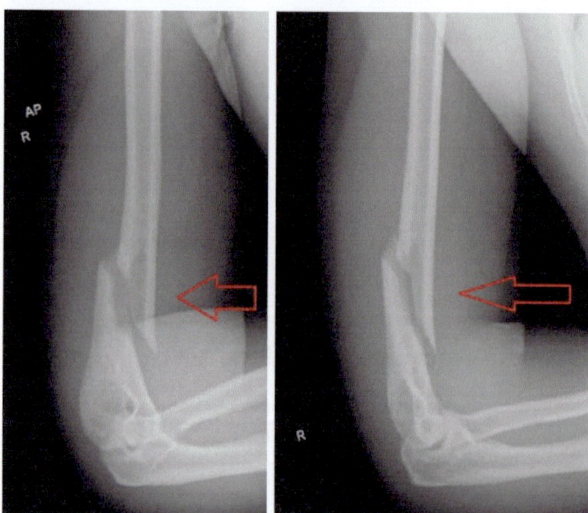

Reference

1. Greenspan A. Orthopedic imaging: a practical approach. 6th ed. Wolters Kluwer; 2015.

Figure 8.1 demonstrates the basic anatomical structures visible on both standard antero-posterior (AP) and axial shoulder x-rays.

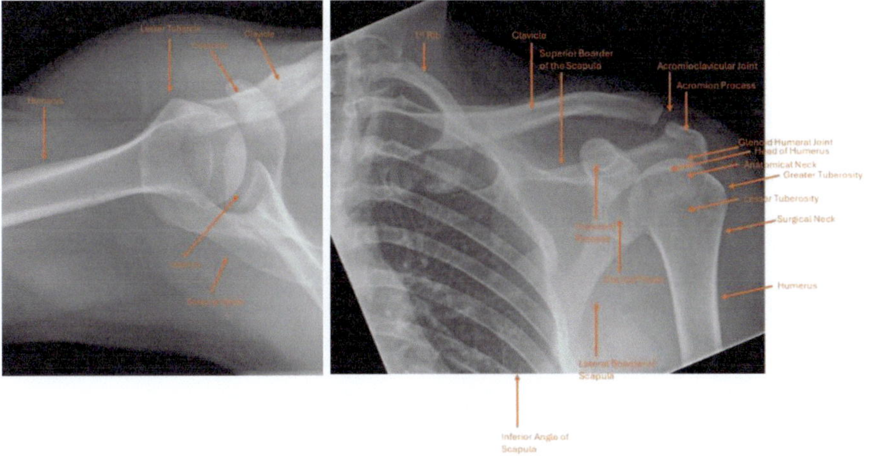

Fig. 8.1 Anatomical structures of the shoulder on the AP and axial views

S. Moughal, *Fracture Finder: A Practical Guide to Interpreting Upper and Lower Limb X-Rays for Radiographers*,
https://doi.org/10.1007/978-3-032-17324-9_8

8.1   Standard Views, Centring Points and Area of Interest

Antero-posterior The affected shoulder should be placed against the erect image receptor, with the torso rotated approximately 15° towards the affected side. This rotation brings the plane of the glenoid fossa perpendicular to the image receptor, allowing improved visualisation of the glenohumeral joint space. The hand should be supinated, and the arm should be slightly abducted away from the body. This positioning helps avoid superimposition of the humeral head by the arm and enables more precise visualisation of the greater tuberosity of the humerus.

The centring point is over the coracoid process.

Axial The image receptor is placed on the tabletop, which is lowered to waist level for patient comfort. The patient's affected arm is abducted over the image receptor. This position allows clear visualisation of the humeral head, glenoid fossa and joint space without overlap. The hand can be supinated or kept in a neutral position. The centring point is over the middle of the glenohumeral joint.

Area of Interest The area of interest in the AP view includes the entire humeral head and proximal humerus. The glenohumeral joint space should be well visualised, along with the glenoid fossa. The lateral aspect of the scapula, acromion, and clavicle should be included. Soft tissues around the shoulder must be visible to assess for swelling or abnormalities. Collimation should be tight to minimise patient dose.

For the axial view, the focus is on the humeral head, glenohumeral joint space and the glenoid fossa. The image should also include the coracoid process and the proximal humerus. The arm should be abducted to avoid the superimposition of structures. Soft tissues must be visible, and collimation should be restricted to the joint area [1].

8.2   General Evaluation of Shoulder Examinations

1. The glenohumeral joint space should be visible, with minimal overlap of the humeral head and glenoid cavity.
2. The greater tuberosity should be seen in profile laterally.
3. The lesser tuberosity should be superimposed over the humeral head medially.
4. The lateral two-thirds of the clavicle, the proximal third of the humerus and the superior scapula should be included within the collimation field.
5. The soft tissue and bony trabecular pattern should be visualised, indicating appropriate exposure.
6. There should be no rotation, demonstrated by the symmetrical appearance of the scapular body and clear glenoid outline.
7. Adequate contrast and sharpness should allow for the assessment of cortical margins and potential pathology.

8.3   Common Shoulder Fracture/Pathologies

8.3.1   Anterior Dislocation of the Glenohumeral Joint (GHJ)

The humeral head is displaced anteriorly and lies in front of the coracoid process, positioned anterior to the glenoid fossa. Figure 8.2 demonstrates the anterior dislocation. It is visualised in both AP and axial views.

8.3.2   Bankart Lesion

This is an avulsion fracture of the anteroinferior glenoid rim (Fig. 8.3). This fracture type is associated with recurrent anterior shoulder dislocations.

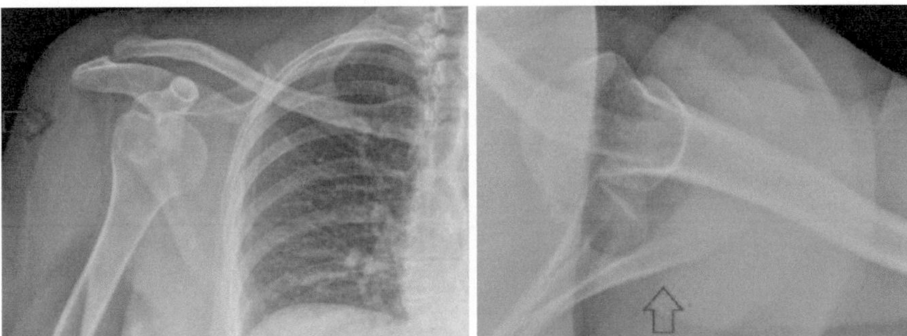

Fig. 8.2   Anterior dislocation of the GHJ

Fig. 8.3   Drawing example of a Bankart lesion

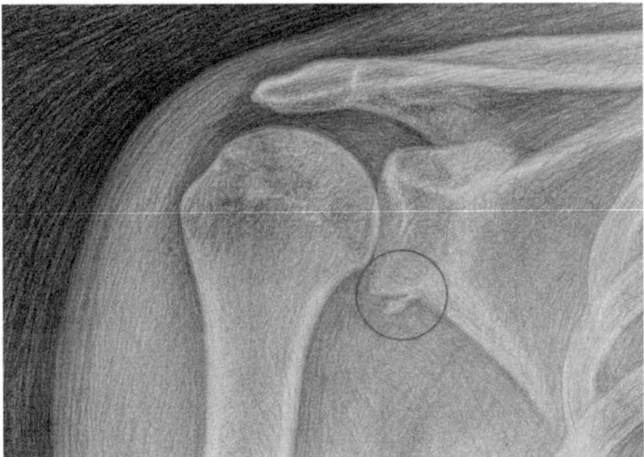

8.3.3 Hill-Sachs Lesion

This is a compression fracture of the posterolateral aspect of the humeral head, which is caused by impaction against the anterior glenoid rim during an anterior dislocation. It is often associated with a Bankart's lesion. This injury is demonstrated in Fig. 8.4.

8.3.4 Posterior Dislocation of the Glenohumeral Joint

The humeral head is displaced posteriorly and lies behind the coracoid process, positioned posterior to the glenoid fossa. This is demonstrated in Fig. 8.5. The humeral head will appear rounded and symmetrical on an AP view—this is commonly known as the 'lightbulb sign'.

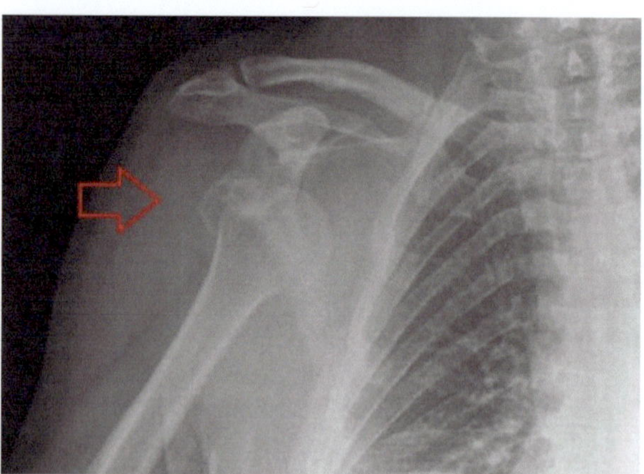

Fig. 8.4 Hill-Sachs lesion

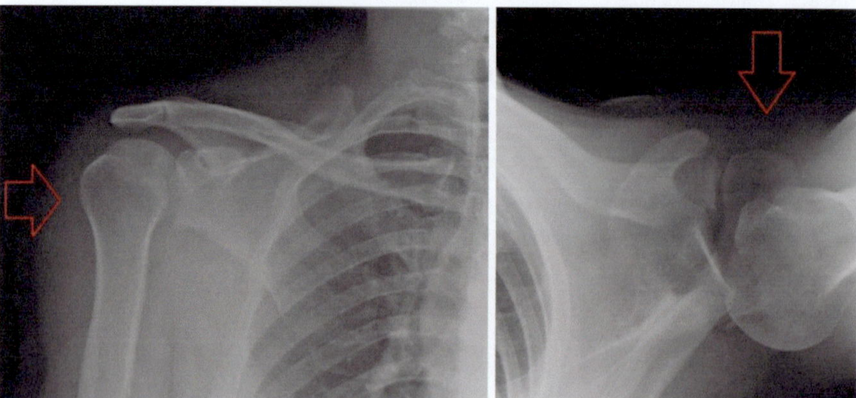

Fig. 8.5 Posterior dislocation of the GHJ

Fig. 8.6 Scapula fracture

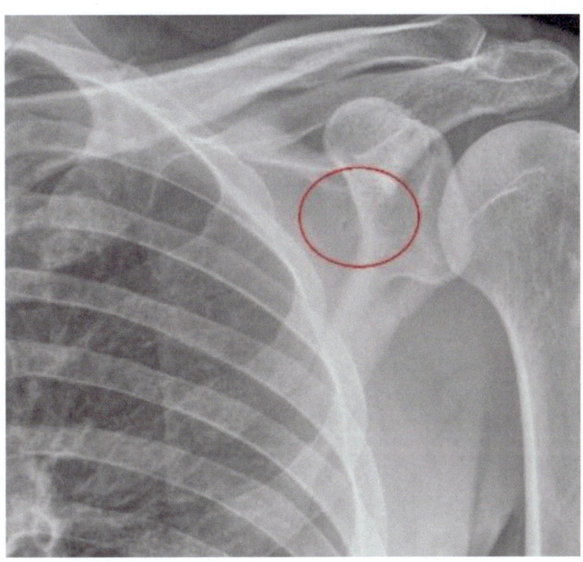

8.3.5 Scapula Fractures

This is a fracture involving the scapula and can occur in any part of its anatomy, including the body, spine, acromion, coracoid or glenoid.

Figure 8.6 demonstrates a fracture at the body of the scapula.

Reference

1. Whitley AS, Jefferson G, Holmes K, Sloane C, Anderson C. Clark's positioning in radiography. 13th ed. CRC Press; 2015.

Clavicle

Figure 9.1 demonstrates the basic anatomical structures visible on a standard antero-posterior (AP) shoulder x-ray.

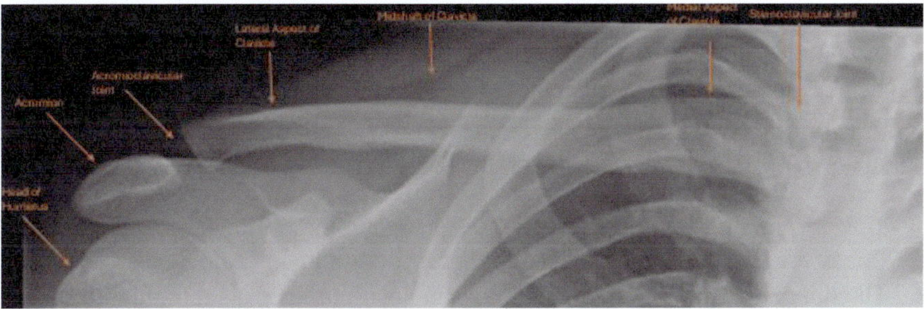

Fig. 9.1 Anatomical structures of the Clavicle on the AP view

9.1   Standard Views, Centring Points and Area of Interest

Antero-Posterior The affected shoulder should be placed against the erect image receptor. The X-ray beam is aimed straight at the middle of the clavicle. The whole clavicle, from the sternoclavicular joint to the acromioclavicular joint, should be included. Arms should hang naturally by the sides to avoid lifting shoulders. Collimate tightly around the clavicle. The centring point is the midshaft of the clavicle.

Axial The affected shoulder should be placed against the erect image receptor. The X-ray beam is angled upward about 15°–30° toward the clavicle. This angle helps see the clavicle clearly above the ribs and shoulder blade. The whole clavicle must be included. Collimate closely around the clavicle. The centring point is the midshaft of the clavicle [1].

9.2   General Evaluation of Clavicle Examinations

1. The entire clavicle should be visible from the sternoclavicular joint medially to the acromioclavicular joint laterally.
2. The clavicle should be well centred on the image receptor, with proper collimation to include the whole bone and reduce patient dose.
3. The cortical outline and trabecular pattern of the clavicle should be sharp and clear, with no motion blur.
4. The surrounding soft tissues should be examined for swelling or signs of injury.
5. Check for fractures, displacement or deformities along the clavicle.
6. The image should be free of artefacts and positioning errors that might obscure critical anatomy.

9.3   Common Clavicle Fracture/Pathologies

9.3.1   Dislocation of the Acromio-Clavicular Joint (ACJ)

The inferior surfaces of the acromion and clavicle should be aligned. The acromio-clavicular (AC) joint space should measure less than 10 mm.

If the joint space exceeds 10 mm as seen in Fig. 9.2, a subluxation or dislocation is likely.

9.3.2   Medial Clavicle Fracture

This is a fracture of the medial third of the clavicle Fig. 9.3, closest to the sternum.

These fractures are uncommon and usually result from high-energy trauma.

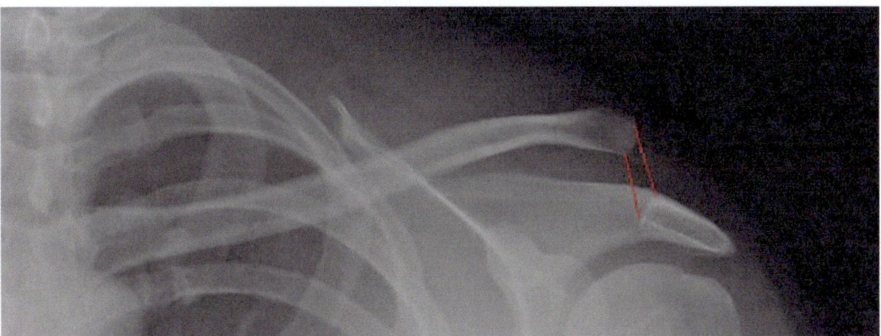

Fig. 9.2   Dislocation of the ACJ

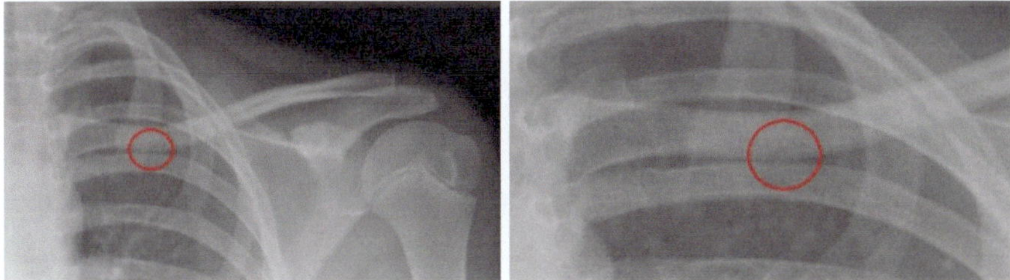

Fig. 9.3   Medial clavicle fracture

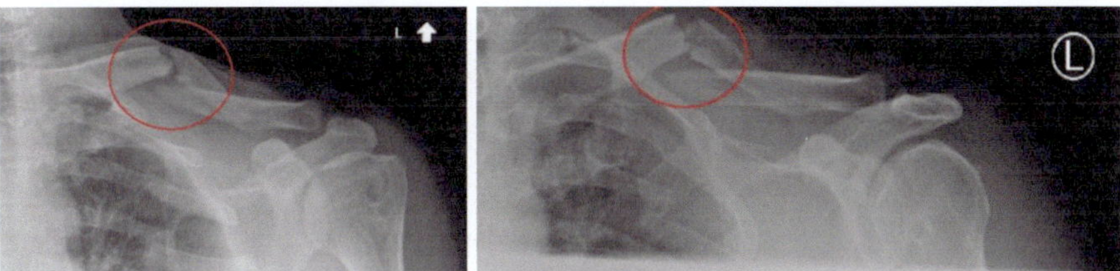

Fig. 9.4   Midshaft clavicle fracture

9.3.3   Midshaft Clavicle Fracture

This is the most common type of clavicle fracture, which involves the middle third of the bone.

The fracture here may be transverse or oblique, usually associated with superior displacement of the medial fragment (Fig. 9.4). These fractures can be angulated and comminuted [2].

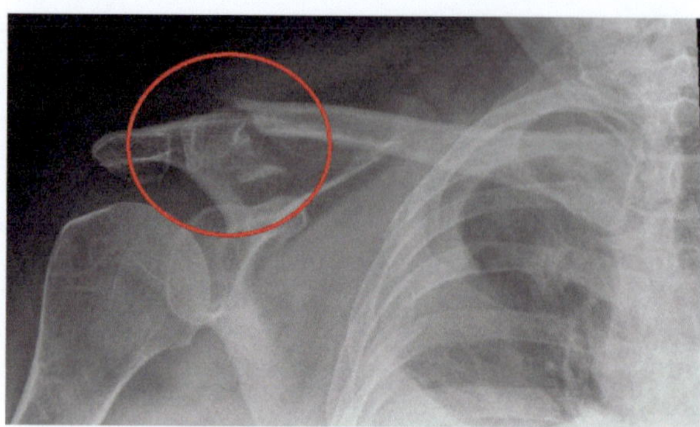

Fig. 9.5 Lateral clavicle fracture

9.3.4   Lateral Clavicle Fracture

This is a fracture seen at the lateral third of the clavicle near the acromioclavicular joint (Fig. 9.5). It is often associated with AC joint disruption.

References

1. Whitley AS, Jefferson G, Holmes K, Sloane C, Anderson C. Clark's positioning in radiography. 13th ed. CRC Press; 2015.
2. Eiff MP, Hatch RL. Fracture management for primary care. 3rd ed. Saunders; 2012.

Part II

Lower Limb Extremity

To accurately comment on, highlight, or identify abnormalities, it is essential to understand the fundamentals, which include being familiar with the standard imaging views and the correct centring points to ensure high-quality diagnostic images.

This chapter will cover the most common pathologies found in the lower limb, including:

  I. Toes/Foot
 II. Ankle
III. Tibia/Fibula
IV. Knee
 V. Femur
VI. Pelvis

It will also outline the standard radiographic views and centring points for each Area.

Figure 10.1 demonstrates the basic anatomical structures visible on both standard Dorsi-Plantar (DP) and oblique toe/foot x-rays.

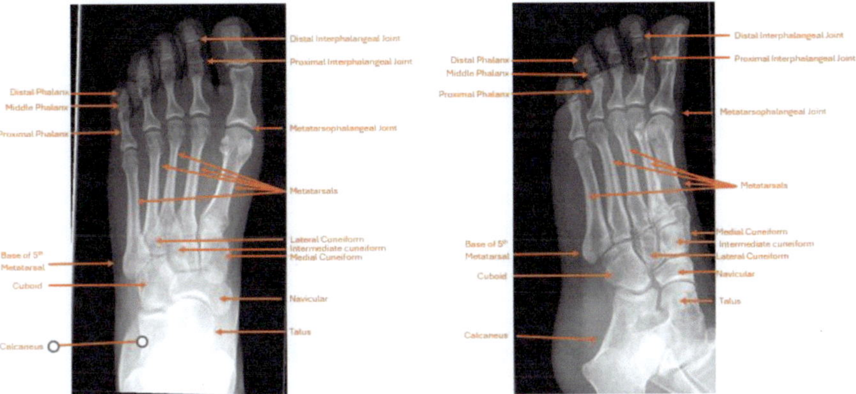

Fig. 10.1 Anatomical structures of the Foot on the DP and oblique views

S. Moughal, *Fracture Finder: A Practical Guide to Interpreting Upper and Lower Limb X-Rays for Radiographers*,
https://doi.org/10.1007/978-3-032-17324-9_10

10.1   Standard Views, Centring Points and Area of Interest

Dorsi-Plantar   The plantar aspect of the foot should be placed flat on the image receptor with the toes extended. When imaging the toes, centre the beam on the interphalangeal joint of the affected toe. When imaging the foot, the beam should be centred over the cuboid–navicular joint (typically around the base of the third metatarsal).

Lateral   Start with the plantar aspect of the foot in contact with the image receptor, then externally rotate the foot until the lateral aspect is in contact with the image receptor. The medial and lateral malleoli should be superimposed. The centring point is over the tubercle of the fifth metatarsal.

Oblique   Start with the plantar aspect of the foot in contact with the image receptor, then medially rotate the foot until it lies at an angle of 30–45° to the image receptor. The centring point is over the cuboid–navicular joint, typically at the base of the third to fifth metatarsals.

Area of Interest   When imaging the toes, collimate to include the affected toe and the adjacent toe. The image should cover from the distal tip of the toe to the distal head of the associated metatarsal.

When imaging the foot, collimate to include from the distal ends of the toes to the base of the ankle joint, including all surrounding soft tissue. This applies to all standard views (DP, oblique and lateral) [1]

10.2   General Evaluation of Toe and Foot Examinations

1. The entire area of interest must be included—for toes, this means the whole digit and associated metatarsal head; for foot exams, all tarsal and metatarsal bones should be visible.
2. The region should be well-centred on the image receptor with correct collimation to reduce dose and include all relevant anatomy.
3. Bone outlines (cortical margins) and internal trabecular patterns should appear sharp, with no evidence of motion blur.
4. Check surrounding soft tissues for swelling, gas or any foreign bodies.
5. Carefully assess all visible joints for alignment, joint space narrowing or widening and possible dislocation or subluxation.
6. Look for fractures (e.g. phalangeal, metatarsal), deformities (e.g. hallux valgus) or signs of trauma to the 5th metatarsal base or Lisfranc region.
7. The image should be free of artefacts or rotation that may affect the accurate evaluation of bone or joint structures.

10.3 Common Toes/Foot Fracture/Pathologies

10.3.1 Unfused Apophysis

This is a secondary ossification centre that has not yet fused with the main bone and is commonly seen running longitudinally lengthwise across the base of the 5th metatarsal (*see* Fig. 10.2). Unfused apophysis appears at the age of 12 for boys and 10 for girls and fuses over the next few years. This can be mistaken for a base of fifth fracture.

10.3.2 Phalangeal Fracture

Fracture of the distal or proximal phalanx is shown in Fig. 10.3. Many types of fractures can occur, such as spiral, transverse and oblique fractures.

10.3.3 Avulsion Fracture

Avulsion fractures in the foot often result from strong ligament or tendon forces pulling a fragment of bone away from its primary structure. These are commonly caused by inversion injuries, twisting or overuse stress.

These are usually found on the lateral aspect of the cuboid, dorsal surface of the navicular and dorsal surface of the talus.

Figure 10.4 shows an avulsion fracture of the cuboid.

Fig. 10.2 Unfused apophysis

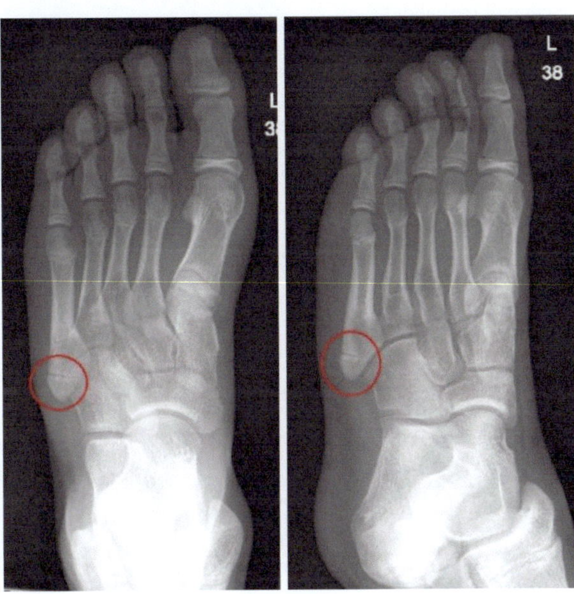

Fig. 10.3 Phalangeal fracture

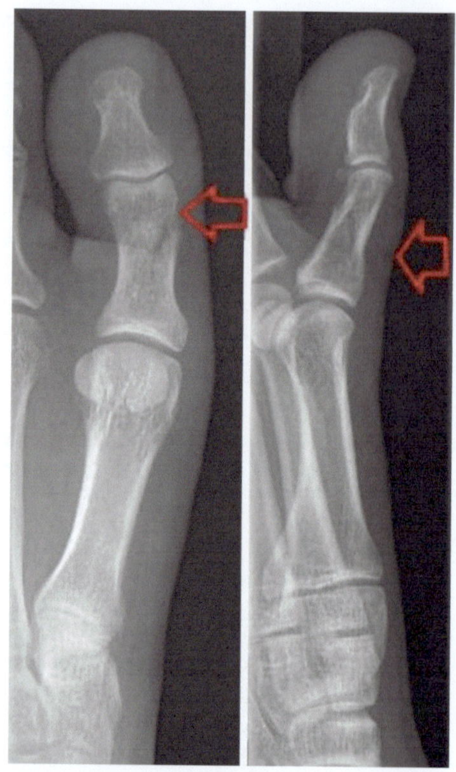

Fig. 10.4 Avulsion fracture of the cuboid

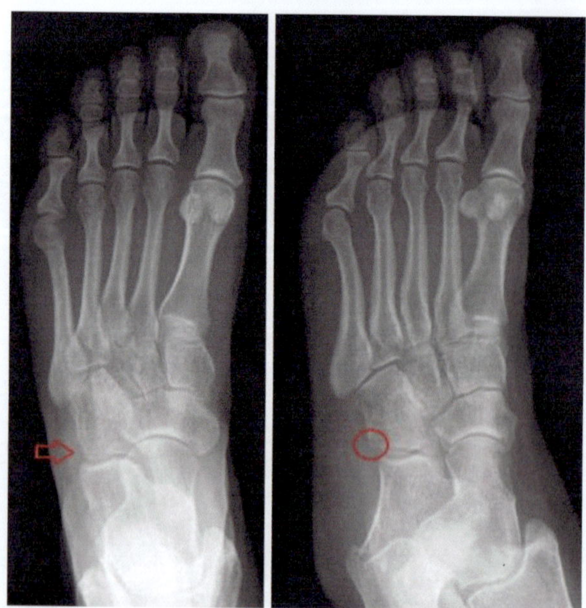

10.3.4 Jones Fracture

This is an extra-articular transverse fracture of the fifth metatarsal (*see* Fig. 10.5). It occurs at the metaphyseal-diaphyseal junction. This fracture is high risk of non-union due to its limited blood supply.

10.3.5 Base of Fifth Fracture

This is a transverse fracture seen at the base of the fifth metatarsal (Fig. 10.6). Avulsion fractures can also occur at the base of the fifth metatarsal, usually involving the metatarsal tuberosity.

10.3.6 Lisfranc Fracture Dislocation

This is a fracture dislocation seen at the tarsometatarsal joints, often affecting the bases of the metatarsals (see Fig. 10.7).

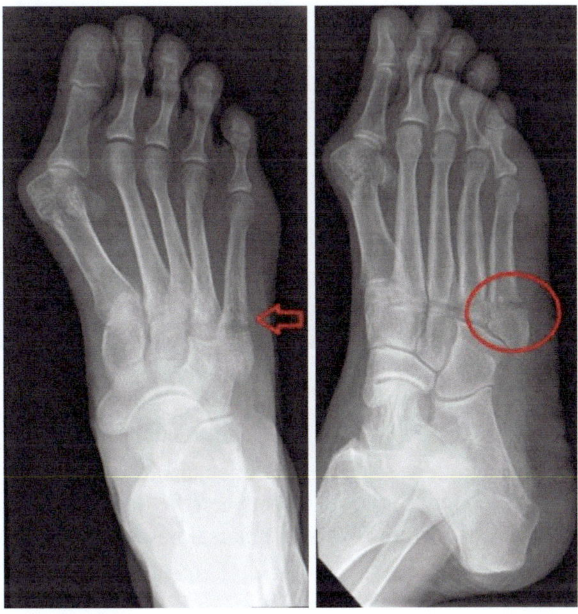

Fig. 10.5 Jones fracture

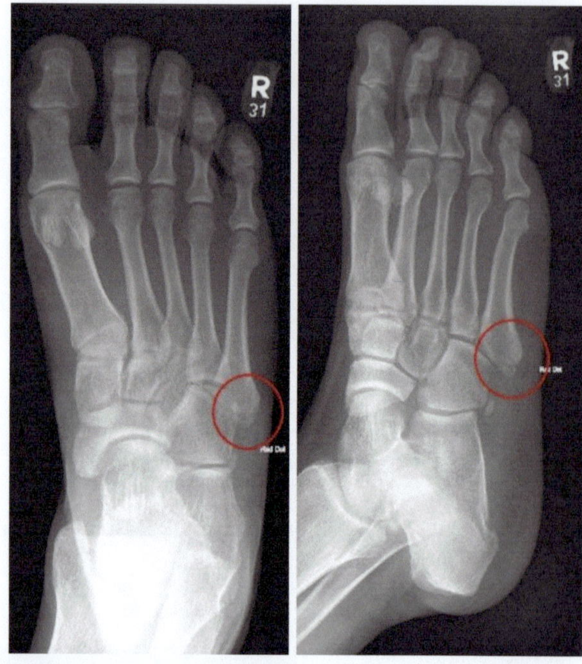

Fig. 10.6 Base of fifth fracture

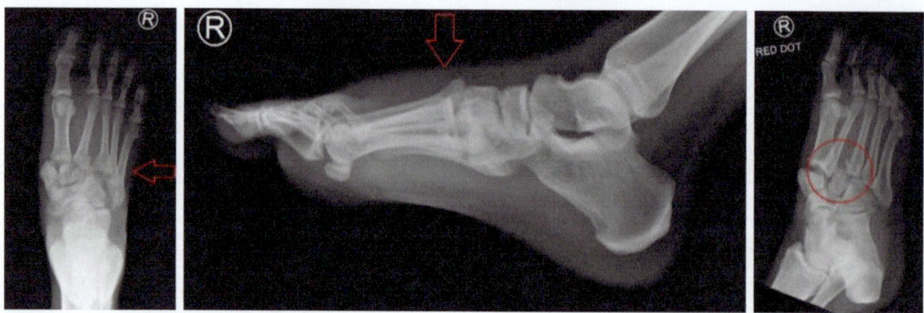

Fig. 10.7 Lisfranc fracture dislocation

Misalignment of the second metatarsal base relating to the middle cuneiform is seen. Widening of the space between the first and second metatarsal may be visual. Associated fractures of the metatarsal bases or cuneiform may occur.

10.3.7 Hallux Valgus

Hallux valgus is a deformity of the first toe where the first metatarsal deviates medially and the hallux points laterally towards the other toes. This condition often causes a visible bunion at the first MTP joint (see Fig. 10.8).

Fig. 10.8 Halux valgus

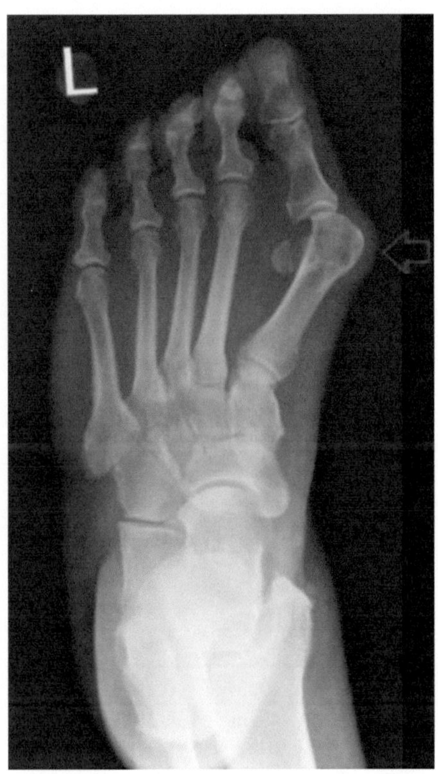

10.3.8 Stress Fracture

A stress fracture is a hairline crack in the bone caused by repetitive strain or overuse, rather than acute trauma (see Fig. 10.9).

Fig. 10.9 Stress fracture

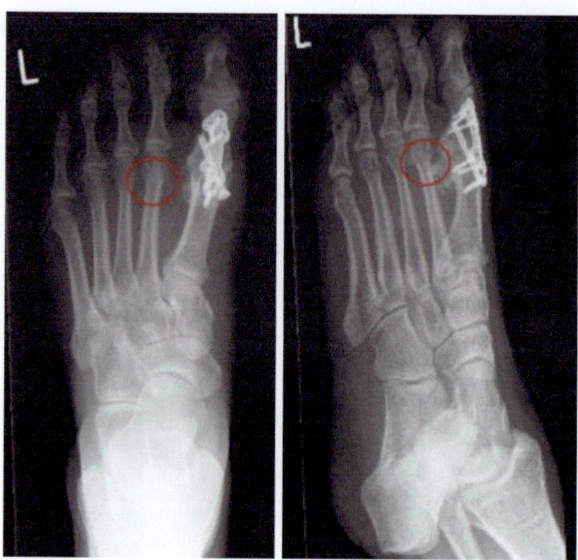

Reference

1. Bontrager KL, Lampignano JP. Textbook of radiographic positioning and related anatomy. 9th ed. Elsevier; 2018.

Ankle

11

Figure 11.1 demonstrates the basic anatomical structures visible on both standard anteroposterior (AP) and lateral ankle x-rays.

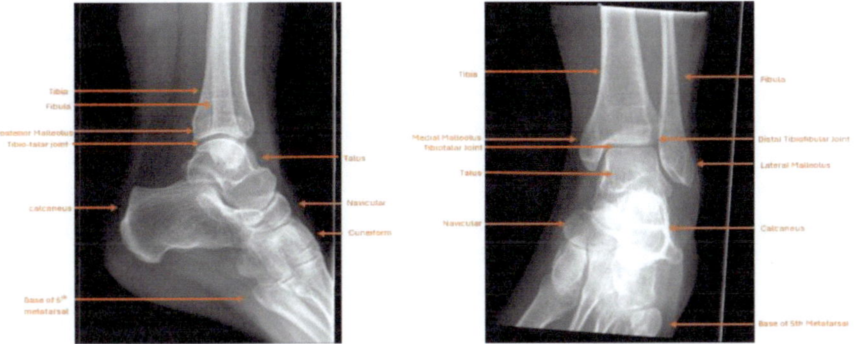

Fig. 11.1 Anatomical structures of the ankle on the AP and lateral views

S. Moughal, *Fracture Finder: A Practical Guide to Interpreting Upper and Lower Limb X-Rays for Radiographers*,
https://doi.org/10.1007/978-3-032-17324-9_11

11.1   Standard Views, Centring Points and Area of Interest

Antero-Posterior The affected ankle should be positioned with the leg extended and on the image receptor. The ankle should be dorsiflexed, allowing the joint space to open. Medially rotate the ankle slightly to achieve a mortise view. The centring point is midway between the medial and lateral malleoli.

Lateral The lateral aspect of the affected ankle should be positioned with the leg extended and on the image receptor. The medial and lateral malleoli should be superimposed with the foot dorsiflexed, allowing the joint space to open up. The centring point is the lateral malleolus.

Area of Interest The distal third of the tib/fib to the base of the fifth should be included in both views [1].

11.2   General Evaluation of Ankle Examinations

1. The image should include the distal third of the tibia and fibula, the ankle joint and the talus (the talar dome should be open).
2. Ensure the ankle joint is well centred on the image receptor, with appropriate collimation to reduce dose and include all required anatomy.
3. Bony cortices and trabecular detail should be visualised with no motion blur or artefact.
4. The joint space should be assessed for symmetry and narrowing, especially at the tibiotalar and distal tibiofibular joints.
5. Evaluate the medial and lateral malleoli, talar dome and posterior malleolus for fractures or irregularities.
6. Inspect soft tissues for signs of swelling, displacement or gas, particularly around the malleoli and anterior joint line.
7. The image should be free from rotation, poor positioning or artefacts that may obscure fracture lines or joint spaces.

Assess Bohrs Angle
Draw two lines along the anterior and posterior edges of the calcaneus.
   A normal angle should be 20 to 40°; any less than this suggests a calcaneus fracture (*see* Fig. 11.2).

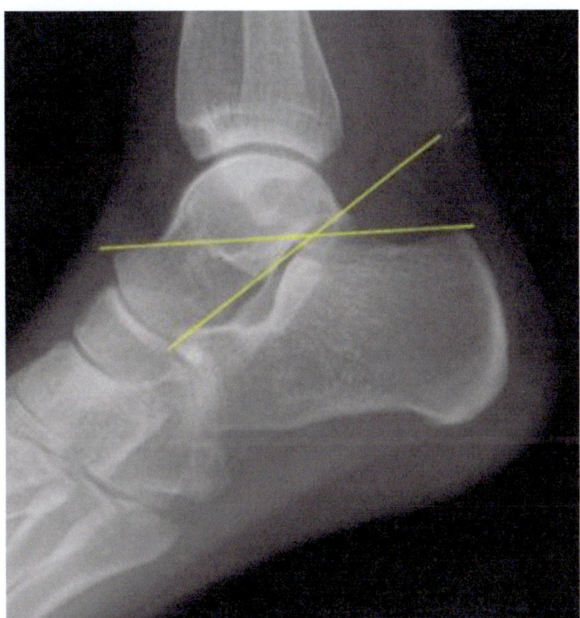

Fig. 11.2 How to assess Bohr's angle

11.3 Common Ankle Fracture/Pathologies

11.3.1 Osteochondral Fracture

This is an avulsion fracture of the talar dome (*see* Fig. 11.3).

11.3.2 Bimalleolar Fracture

This is a fracture that involves two out of the three malleoli: usually the medial malleolus and the lateral malleolus (*see* Fig. 11.4). This fracture type typically affects the ankle joint and is therefore classified as an intra-articular fracture.

11.3.3 Trimalleolar Fracture

This is a fracture that involves all three malleoli: medial, lateral and posterior (this is the posterior aspect of the distal tibia (*see* Fig. 11.5). This fracture type typically affects the ankle joint and is therefore classified as an intra-articular fracture.

Fig. 11.3 Osteochondral fracture

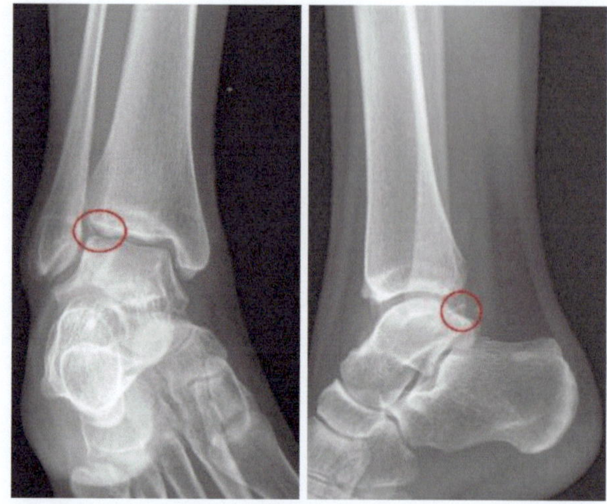

Fig. 11.4 Bimalleolar fracture

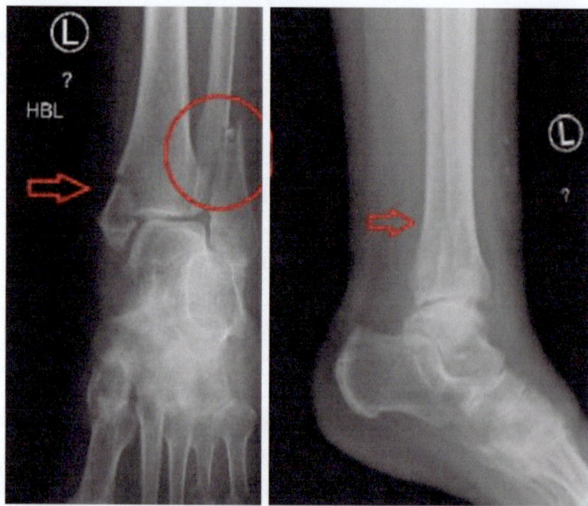

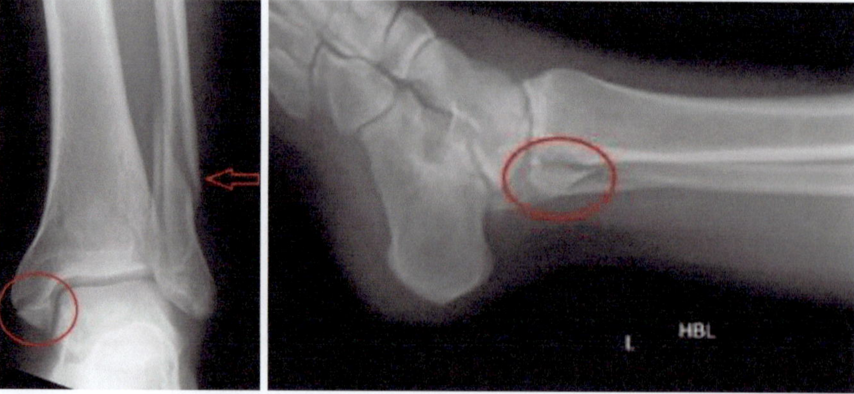

Fig. 11.5 Trimalleolar fracture

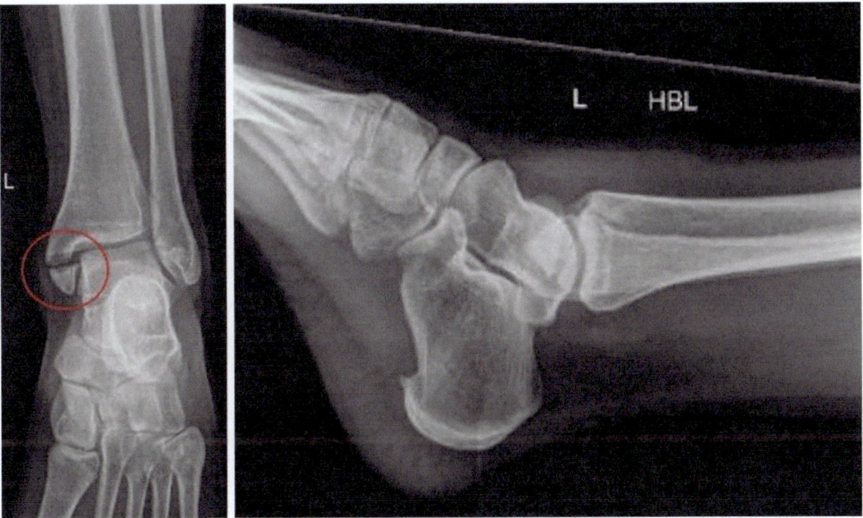

Fig. 11.6 Medial malleolar fracture

11.3.4 Medial Malleolar Fracture

This is an isolated fracture of the medial malleolus (*see* Fig. 11.6), the bony prominence on the inner aspect of the ankle (part of the distal tibia). A fracture of the medial malleolus can be non-displaced or displaced, with displaced fractures often requiring surgical intervention [2]

11.3.5 Lateral Malleolar Fracture

This is a fracture of the lateral malleolus (*see* Fig. 11.7), which is the distal end of the fibula. It can occur as an isolated injury or be part of a bimalleolar or trimalleolar fracture. A fracture of the lateral malleolus can be displaced or non-displaced. Displaced fractures may require surgery.

11.3.6 Calcaneum Fracture

This is a fracture of the calcaneus (*see* Fig. 11.8), typically caused by high-impact trauma, such as a fall from a height. It can be intra-articular (involving the subtalar joint) or extra-articular. These fractures can be displaced and often require CT imaging for full assessment.

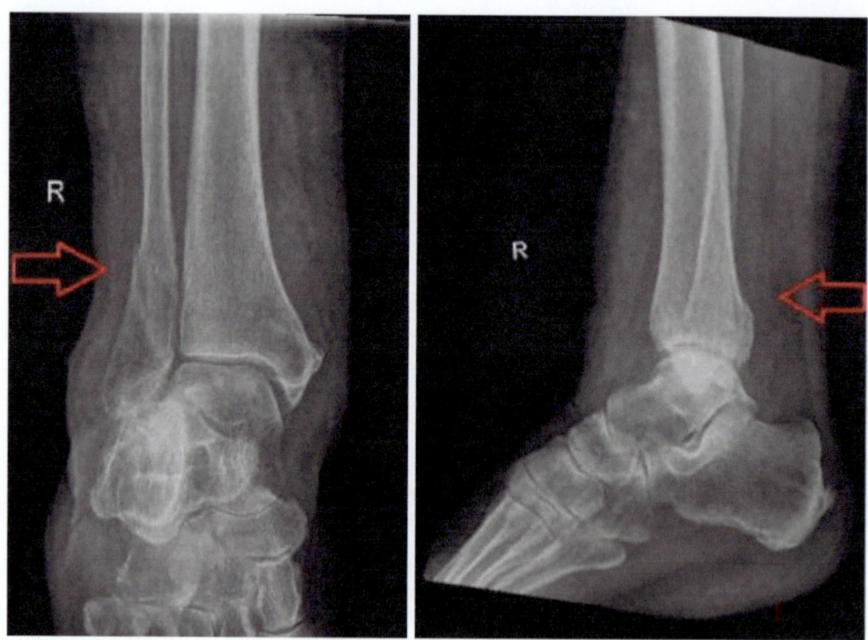

Fig. 11.7 Lateral malleolar fracture

Fig. 11.8 Calcaneum fracture

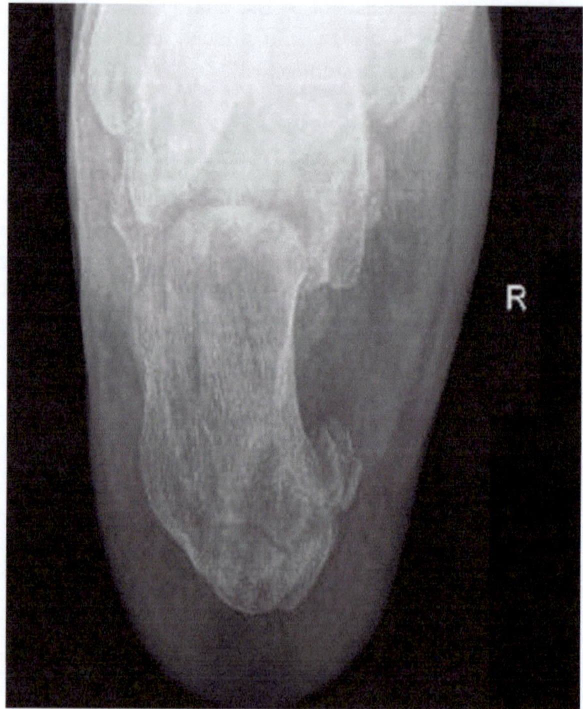

11.3.7 Salter Harris Fracture

This is a fracture that involves the growth plate (physis) in children. It can affect future bone growth depending on the type. There are five main types:

- Type I – fracture through the growth plate only (*see* Fig. 11.9).
- Type II – through the growth plate and metaphysis (*see* Fig. 11.10).
- Type III – through the growth plate and epiphysis (*see* Fig. 11.11).
- Type IV – through the metaphysis, growth plate, and epiphysis (*see* Fig. 11.12).
- Type V – compression injury to the growth plate (*see* Fig. 11.13).

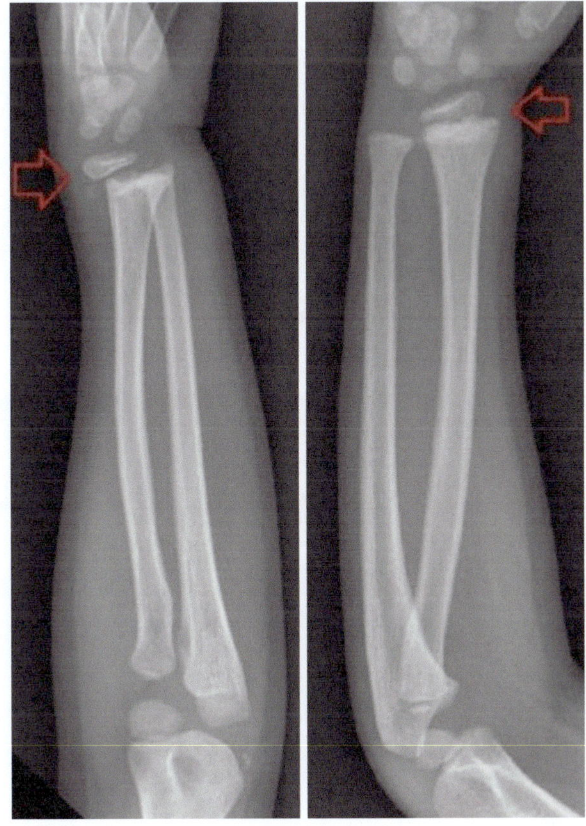

Fig. 11.9 Salter-Harris fracture type I

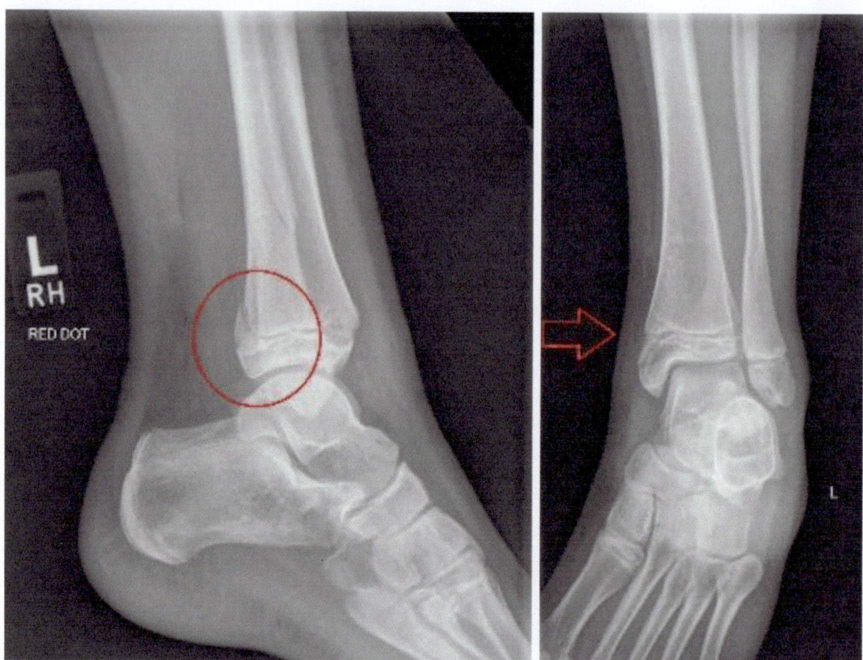

Fig. 11.10 Salter-Harris fracture type II

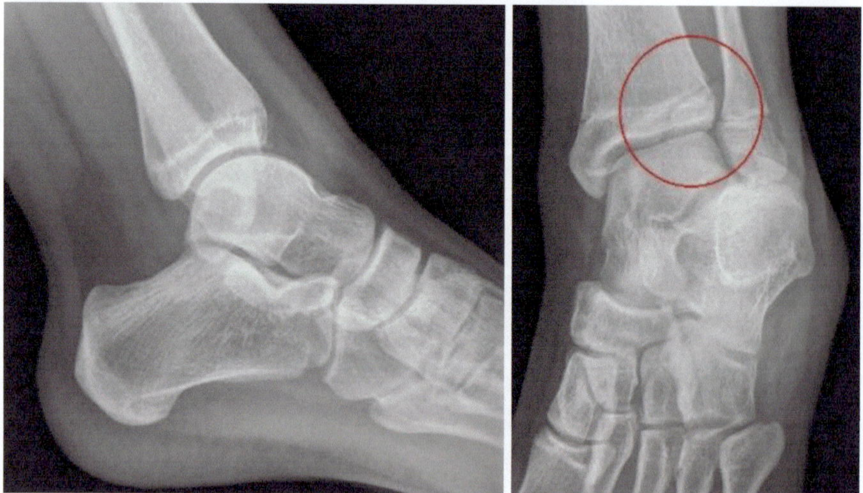

Fig. 11.11 Salter-Harris fracture type III

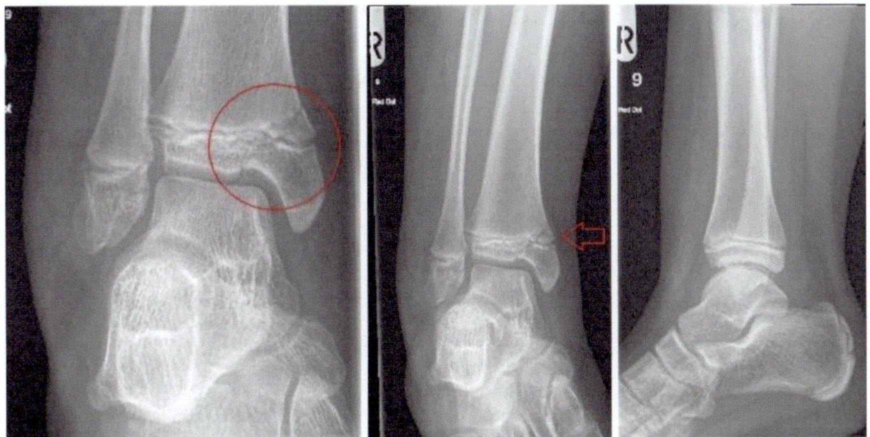

Fig. 11.12 Salter-Harris fracture type IV

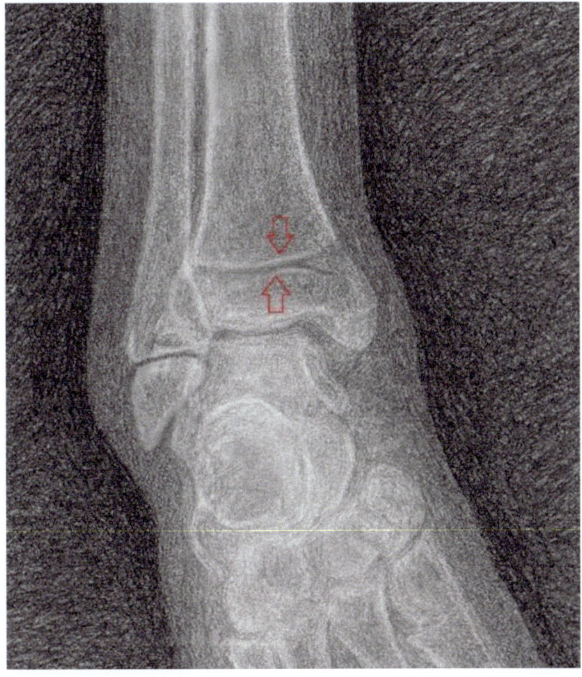

Fig. 11.13 Salter-Harris fracture type V

References

1. Whitley AS, Jefferson G, Holmes K, Sloane C, Anderson C. Clark's positioning in radiography. 13th ed. CRC Press; 2015.
2. Eiff MP, Hatch RL. Fracture management for primary care. 3rd ed. Saunders; 2012.

Tibia/Fibula 12

Figure 12.1 demonstrates the basic anatomical structures visible on both standard anteroposterior (AP) and lateral tibia/fibula x-rays.

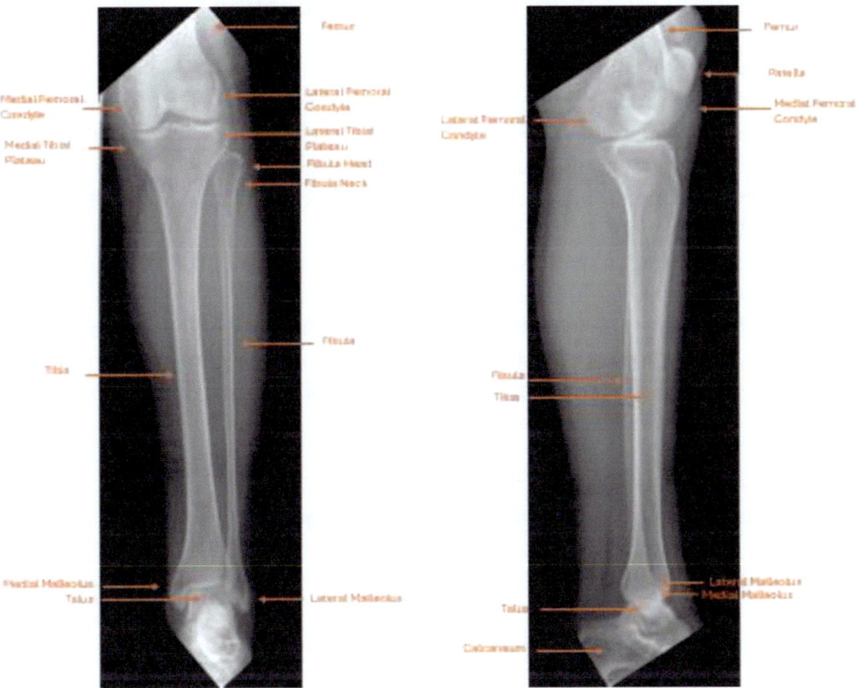

Fig. 12.1 Anatomical structures of the tibia/fibular on the AP and lateral views

S. Moughal, *Fracture Finder: A Practical Guide to Interpreting Upper and Lower Limb X-Rays for Radiographers*,
https://doi.org/10.1007/978-3-032-17324-9_12

12.1   Standard Views, Centring Points and Area of Interest

Anteroposterior   Supine on the table with the affected leg extended over the image receptor, ensuring the posterior aspect of the leg is in contact. The leg should be slightly internally rotated to ensure the malleoli are equidistant. The centring point is midway between the knee and ankle joint.

Lateral   Supine on the table with the leg extended and the posterior aspect in contact with the image receptor initially. Then, externally rotate the affected leg so that the lateral aspect is in complete contact with the receptor. The medial and lateral malleoli should be superimposed. The centring point is placed midway between the knee and ankle joints.

Area of Interest   The entire tibia and fibula should be included, with the knee and ankle joint visualised. The surrounding soft tissue should also be included [1].

12.2   General Evaluation of Tib/Fib Examinations

1. The entire length of the tibia and fibula must be included, from the knee joint proximally to the ankle joint distally.
2. The tibia and fibula should be centred on the image receptor with proper collimation to include both joints and reduce unnecessary exposure.
3. The cortical outline and internal trabecular pattern of both bones should be sharp, with no motion artefact.
4. Both the knee and ankle joints should be visible to assess for alignment, joint effusion or extension of fractures.
5. Evaluate for fractures, angulation, displacement or rotation of the tibia and fibula.
6. Inspect surrounding soft tissues for swelling, gas or signs of open fracture.
7. The image should be free from artefacts or rotation that could obscure pathology or alter anatomical appearance.

12.3   Common Tib/Fib Fracture/Pathologies

12.3.1 Tibial Fracture

This is a fracture of the tibia, which can occur at any part of the bone but is most commonly seen at the midshaft (*see* Fig. 12.2). As a long bone, the tibia can present with various fracture patterns, including spiral, oblique or transverse. These fractures can be caused by direct trauma, twisting injuries or high-impact forces like road traffic accidents or falls.

Fig. 12.2 Tibial fracture

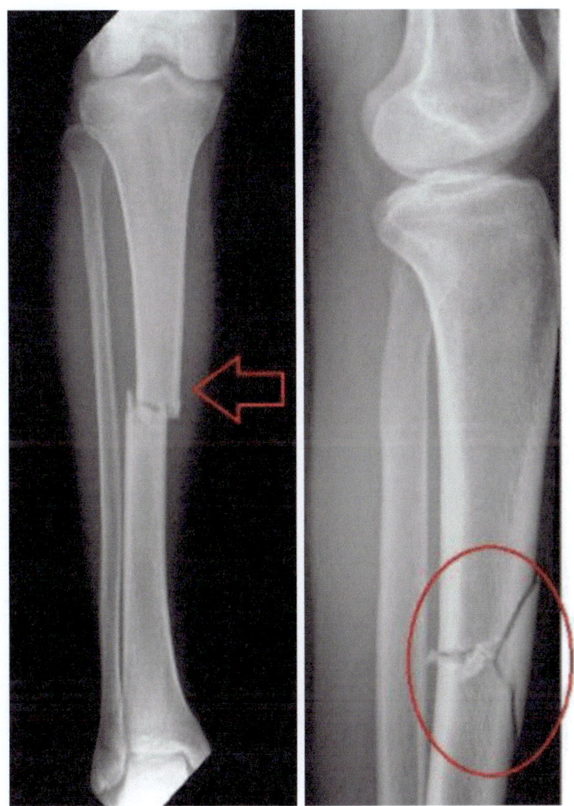

12.3.2 Toddlers Fracture

This is a spiral fracture of the distal tibia commonly seen in young children, usually under 3 years old. It often occurs after a low energy fall or twisting injury (*see* Fig. 12.3).

12.3.3 Maisonneuve Fracture

This is a fracture of the proximal fibula, accompanied by a fracture of the medial malleolus. The tibiofibular joint space may show some widening due to ligamentous injury (*see* Fig. 12.4) [2].

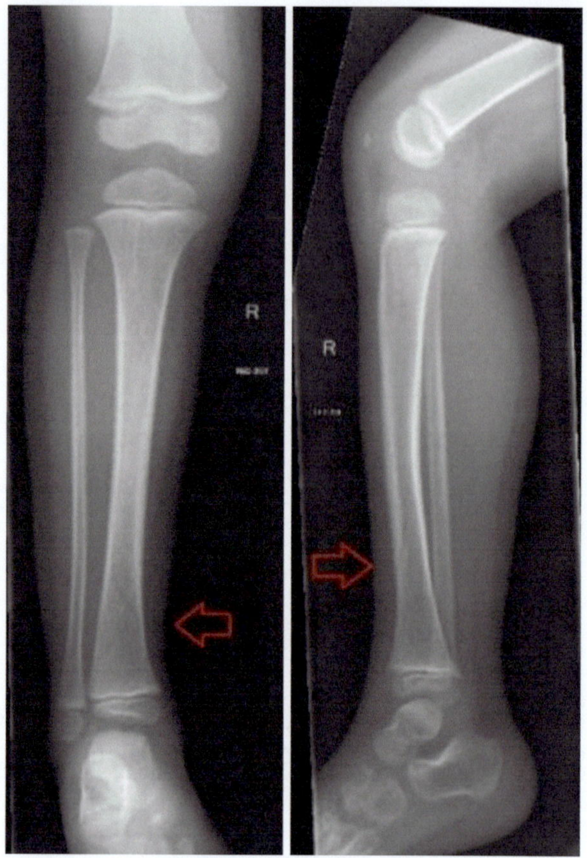

Fig. 12.3 Toddlers fracture

The tibia and fibula form a ring-like structure with the distal and proximal tibiofibular joints. Because of this structure, a fracture in one part of the ring often indicates another injury elsewhere in the ring. This is why it is important to assess the entire lower leg, including both tibiofibular joints, for additional fractures if one is identified.

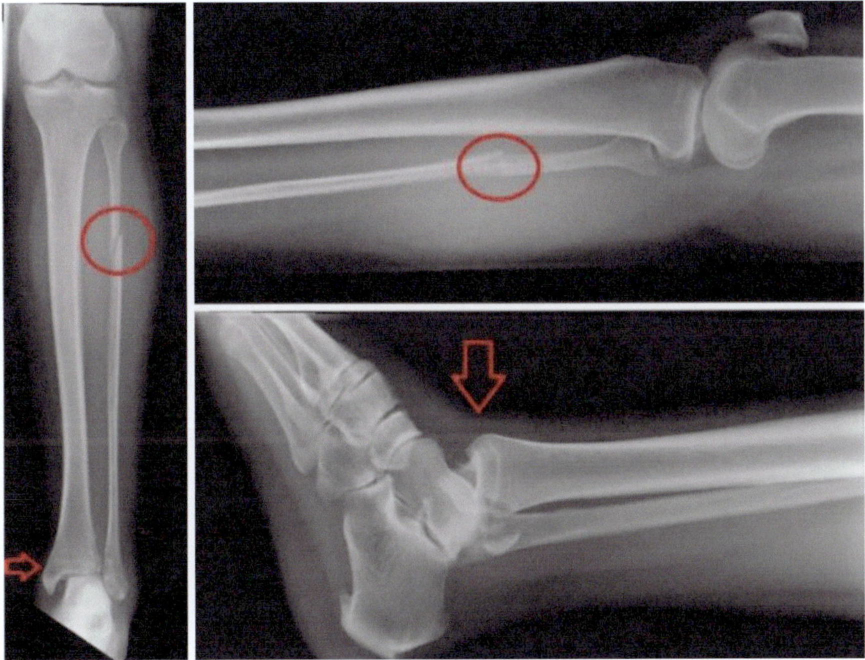

Fig. 12.4 Maisonneuve fracture

References

1. Whitley AS, Jefferson G, Holmes K, Sloane C, Anderson C. Clark's positioning in radiography. 13th ed. CRC Press; 2015.
2. Eiff MP, Hatch RL. Fracture management for primary care. 3rd ed. Saunders; 2012.

Knee

13

Figure 13.1 demonstrates the basic anatomical structures visible on both standard anteroposterior (AP) and lateral knee x-rays.

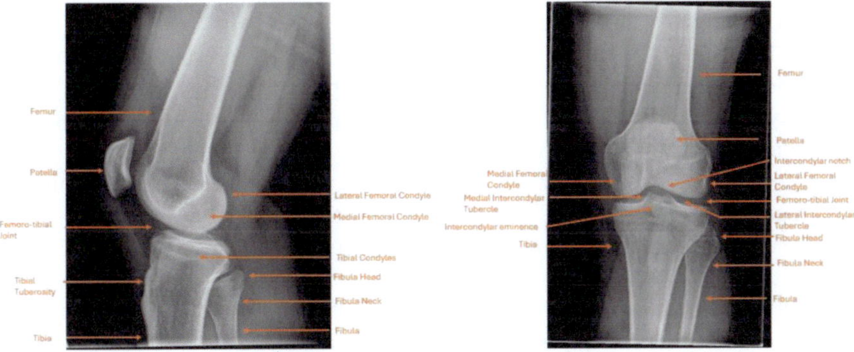

Fig. 13.1 Anatomical structures of the knee on the AP and lateral views

© The Author(s), under exclusive license to Springer Nature Switzerland AG 2026

S. Moughal, *Fracture Finder: A Practical Guide to Interpreting Upper and Lower Limb X-Rays for Radiographers*,

https://doi.org/10.1007/978-3-032-17324-9_13

13.1   Standard Views, Centring Points and Area of Interest

Antero-Posterior   The posterior aspect of the knee should be in contact with the image receptor. The knee is then slightly medially rotated to ensure the patella is positioned centrally. The centring point is below the apex of the patella.

Lateral   Supine on the table with the leg flexed at the knee joint about 45° and the lateral aspect in contact with the image receptor. The femoral condyles should be superimposed. The centring point is the middle of the superior borders of the medial tibial condyle.

Area of Interest   The distal third of the femur and the proximal third of the tibia/ fib should be included with lateral skin borders in view.

13.2   General Evaluation of Knee Examinations

1. The entire knee joint should be included, from the distal femur to the proximal tibia and fibula, as well as the patella [1].
2. The knee should be well centred on the image receptor, with correct collimation to include surrounding soft tissues and reduce patient dose.
3. Bony cortices and trabecular patterns should appear sharp with no evidence of motion or positioning artefact.
4. Assess the joint space between the femur and tibia for narrowing, widening or irregularities.
5. Evaluate the patellofemoral joint for alignment or signs of dislocation or subluxation.
6. Check for fractures, cortical disruption or joint effusion—particularly around the femoral condyles, tibial plateau, fibular head and patella.
7. Soft tissues around the joint, including suprapatellar and infrapatellar areas, should be examined for swelling or displacement.
8. The image should be free from rotation or artefacts that could obscure the joint margins or surrounding anatomy.

13.3   Common Knee Fracture/Pathologies

13.3.1   Arcuate Sign

The arcuate sign is a small fracture seen on knee X-rays at the fibular head (the bone just below the knee on the outer side) (*see* Fig. 13.2). It happens when the ligament called the arcuate ligament pulls a piece of bone off.

This injury typically indicates damage to the back of the knee and the outer part of the knee, which can cause the knee to become unstable.

Fig. 13.2 Arcuate sign

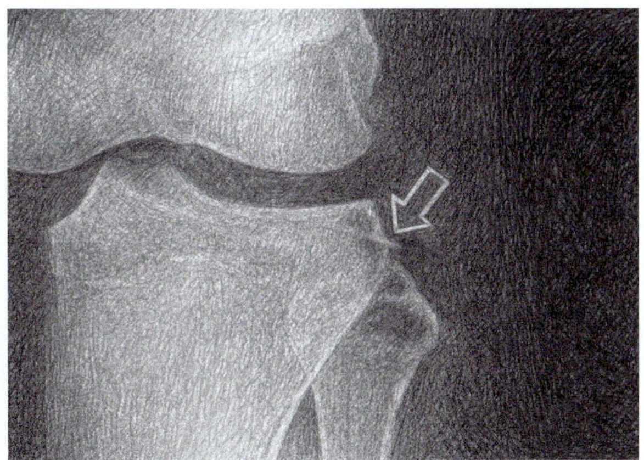

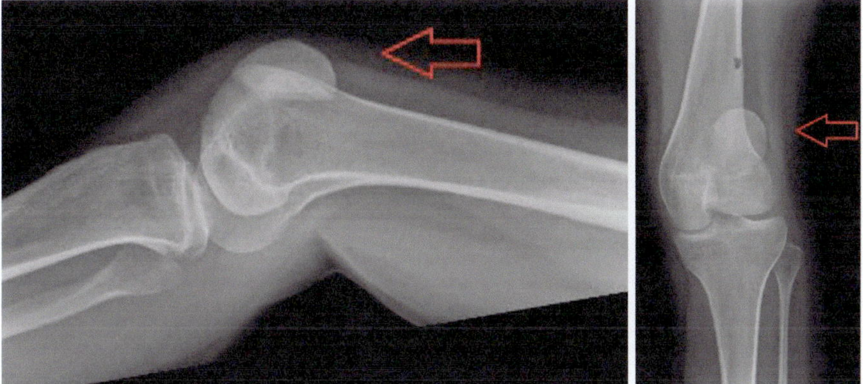

Fig. 13.3 Patella dislocation

13.3.2 Patella Dislocation

This occurs when there is a loss of alignment between the patella and the femur, with the patella sitting outside its central track. In common injuries, the patella is laterally displaced from the trochlear groove of the distal femur; however, some injuries may cause the patella to become medially displaced (*see* Fig. 13.3).

13.3.3 Patella Fracture

Patella fractures are usually seen on the lateral view. The most common fracture seen on the patella is a transverse fracture, which runs horizontally across the bone (*see* Fig. 13.4).

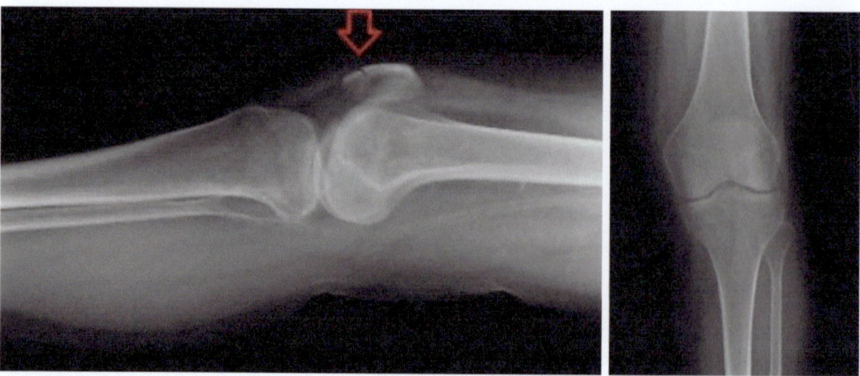

Fig. 13.4   Patella fracture

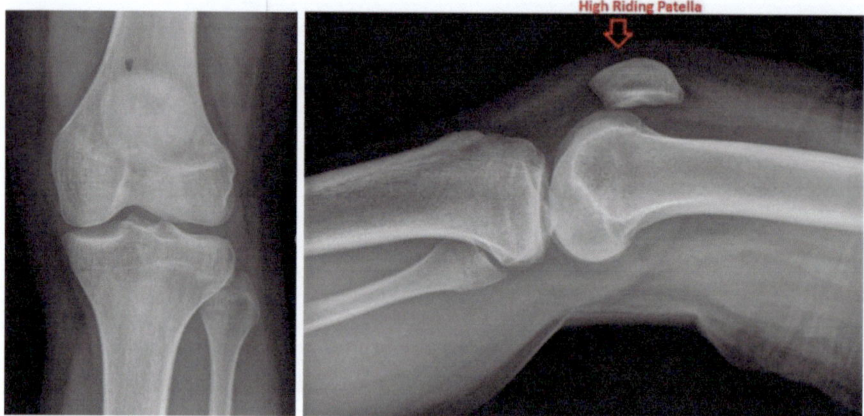

Fig. 13.5   Patella tendon disruption

13.3.4 Patella Tendon Disruption

The patella tendon extends from the inferior pole of the patella to the tibial tuberosity. Typically, the length and tension of the tendon maintain proper patellar position. If the tendon is disrupted or ruptured, it may appear abnormally elongated or discontinuous on imaging, resulting in a high-riding patella due (*see* Fig. 13.5) to the loss of normal tension.

13.3.5 Anterior Cruciate Ligaments (ACL) Fracture

This is a key ligament that supports the knee; it connects the femur to the tibia. An avulsion fracture can occur at the tibial eminence (*see* Fig. 13.6), which is where the ACL attaches.

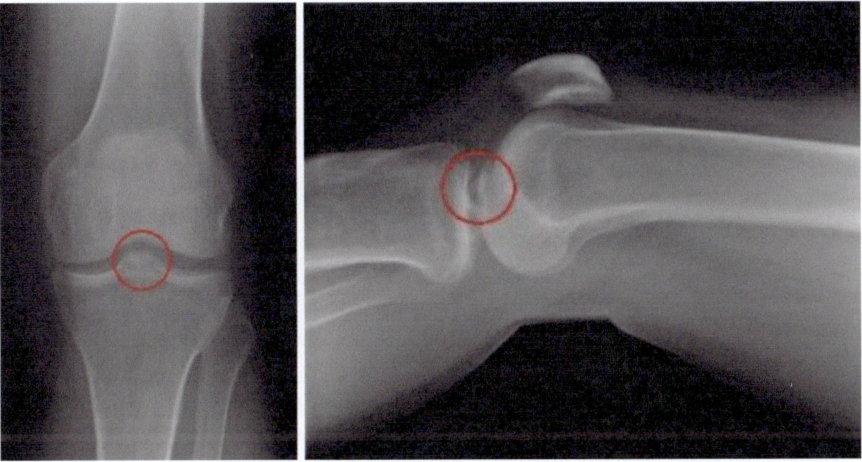

Fig. 13.6 ACL fracture

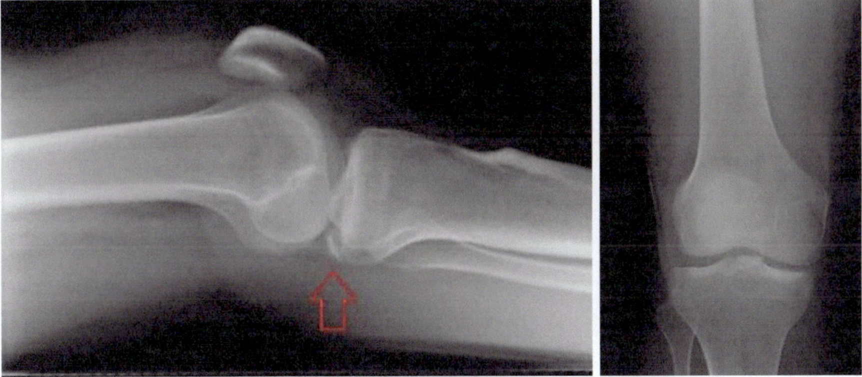

Fig. 13.7 PCL fracture

13.3.6 Posterior Cruciate Ligament (PCL) Fracture

The posterior cruciate ligament (PCL) is another key ligament that supports the knee joint. It runs behind the anterior cruciate ligament (ACL) and connects the femur to the posterior aspect of the tibia. A PCL avulsion fracture can occur at the point where the ligament inserts onto the posterior tibial plateau (*see* Fig. 13.7), typically resulting from direct trauma or hyperflexion injuries.

13.3.7 Bipartite Patella

This is a congenital condition that occurs when the patella does not fuse but instead remains as two separate bones (*see* Fig. 13.8).

It can be mistaken for a patella fracture.

13.3.8 Tibial Plateau Fracture

This is a fracture in the proximal tibia that involves the articular surface of the knee joint. It can affect either the medial or lateral tibial plateau (*see* Fig. 13.9), depending on the mechanism of injury. These fractures can affect joint stability and are often accompanied by ligament or meniscal injuries [2].

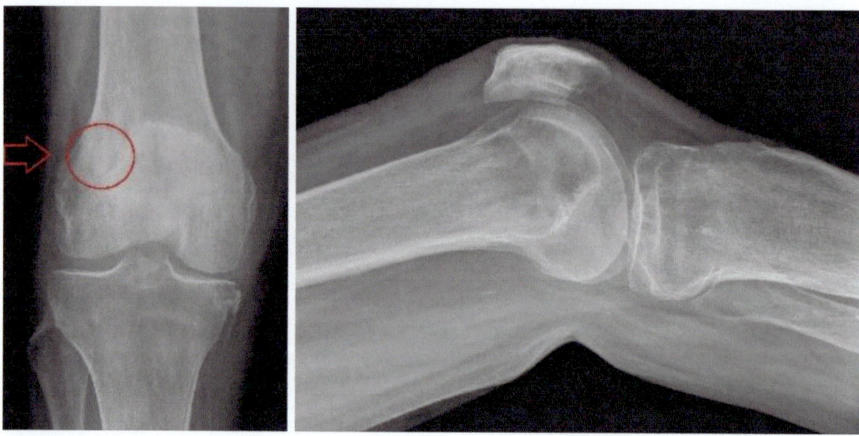

Fig. 13.8 Bipartite fracture

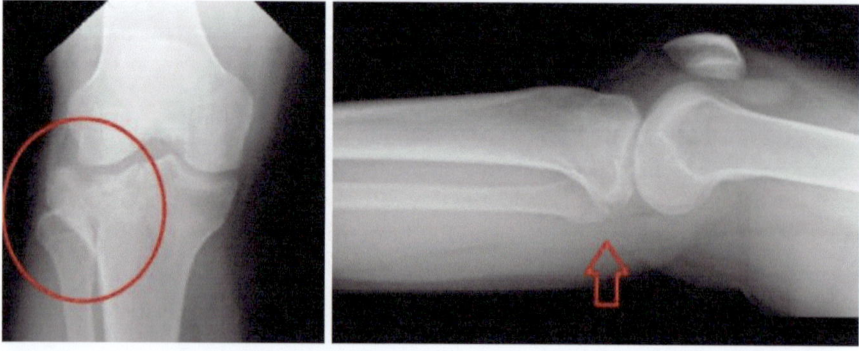

Fig. 13.9 Showing a lateral tibial plateau fracture

13.3.9 Bicondylar Tibial Plateau Fracture

This is a fracture involving both the medial and lateral tibial plateaus (*see* Fig. 13.10).

13.3.10 Segond Fracture

This is a small avulsion fracture on the lateral aspect of the tibial plateau. It is often seen with ACL injuries (*see* Fig. 13.11).

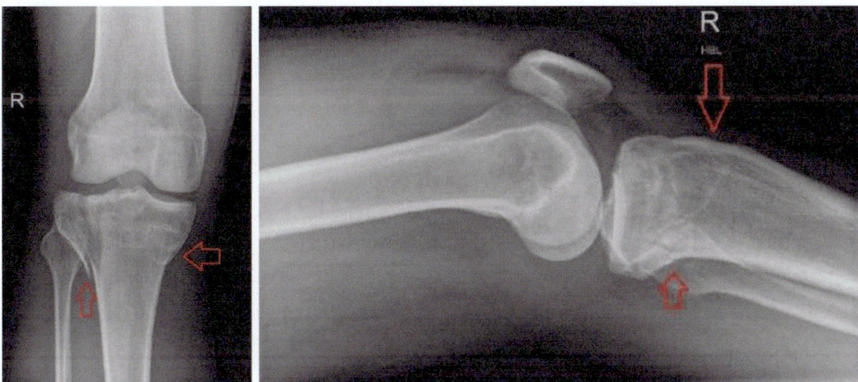

Fig. 13.10 Bicondylar tibial plateau fracture

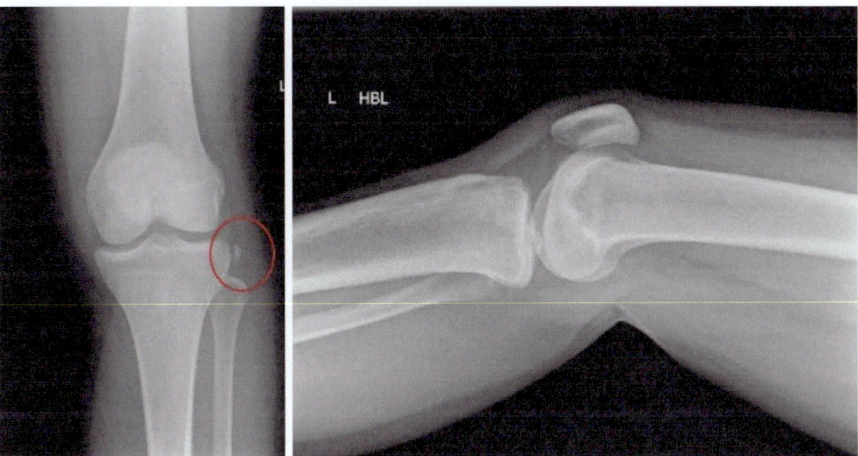

Fig. 13.11 Segond fracture

13.3.11 Reverse Segond Fracture

This is a small avulsion fracture on the medial aspect of the tibial plateau (*see* Fig. 13.12), opposite to a classic Segond fracture. It is often associated with injuries to the posterior cruciate ligament (PCL) and the medial meniscus.

13.3.12 Osgood-Schlatter Disease

Osgood-Schlatter disease is an inflammation where the patellar ligament attaches to the tibial tuberosity (*see* Fig. 13.13). It typically affects active children and teenagers, especially during periods of rapid growth.

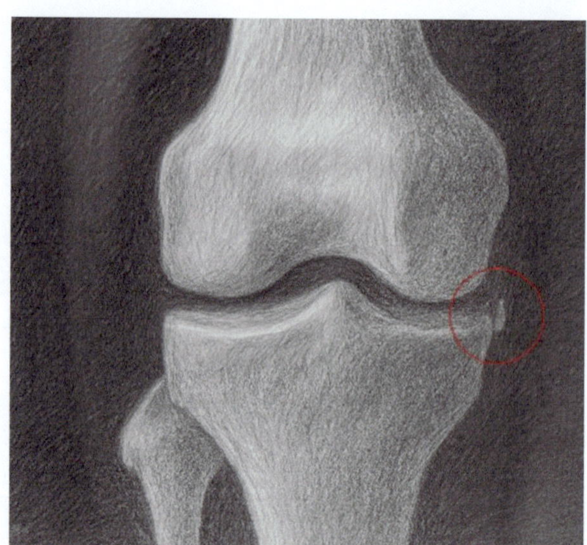

Fig. 13.12 Reverse Segond fracture

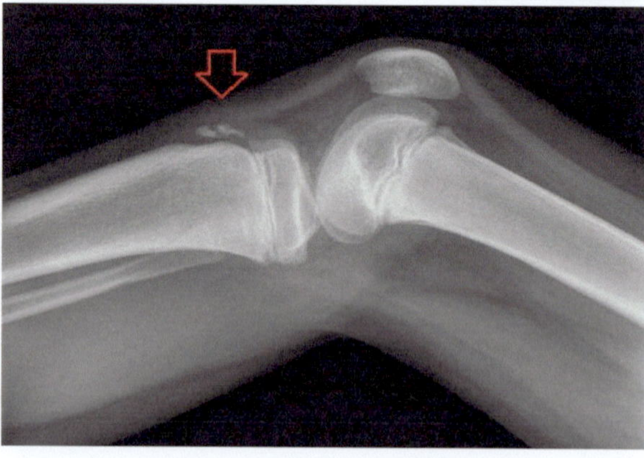

Fig. 13.13 Osgood-Schlatter disease

It is caused by repeated stress or pulling on the growth plate at the top of the shin bone, often from running or jumping. This can lead to pain, swelling and a bony lump just below the knee.

References

1. Bontrager KL, Lampignano JP. Textbook of radiographic positioning and related anatomy. 9th ed. Elsevier; 2018.
2. Greenspan A. Orthopedic imaging: a practical approach. 6th ed. Wolters Kluwer; 2015.

Femur

14

14.1 Standard Views, Centring Points and Area of Interest

Antero-Posterior Supine on the table with the affected leg extended over the image receptor, ensuring the posterior aspect of the femur is in contact. The femoral condyles should be equidistant. The centring point is the midshaft of the femur, midway between the hip and knee joint.

Lateral Supine on the table with the leg extended and the posterior aspect in contact with the image receptor initially. Then, externally rotate to the affected side so that the lateral aspect is in complete contact with the receptor. The knee is flexed with the opposite limbs moved out of the field of view. The femoral condyles should be superimposed. The centring point is at the midshaft of the femur.

Area of Interest The entire femur should be included from the hip joint to the knee joint, with the medial and lateral skin borders included [1].

14.2 General Evaluation of Femur Examinations

1. The entire femur must be included—from the hip joint proximally to the knee joint distally.
2. The femur should be well centred on the image receptor with appropriate collimation to include both joints and reduce patient dose.
3. Bony cortices and trabecular detail should be visualised, with no motion blur or artefacts.
4. Assess for fractures, angulation, displacement or cortical irregularities throughout the femoral shaft.
5. Evaluate both the hip and knee joints for involvement or extension of injury.

© The Author(s), under exclusive license to Springer Nature Switzerland AG 2026
S. Moughal, *Fracture Finder: A Practical Guide to Interpreting Upper and Lower Limb X-Rays for Radiographers*,
https://doi.org/10.1007/978-3-032-17324-9_14

6. The soft tissues surrounding the femur should be examined for swelling, gas or signs of open injury.
7. The image should be free from rotation, poor exposure or positioning errors that could affect the evaluation of the bone or joints.

14.3   Common Femur Fracture/Pathologies

Figure 14.1 illustrates the various types of fractures and indicates where each type commonly occurs along the bone [2].

14.3.1 Capital Fracture

This is an intracapsular fracture seen at the proximal end of the head of the femur. The yellow-highlighted area in Fig. 14.1 demonstrates here capital fractures are found.

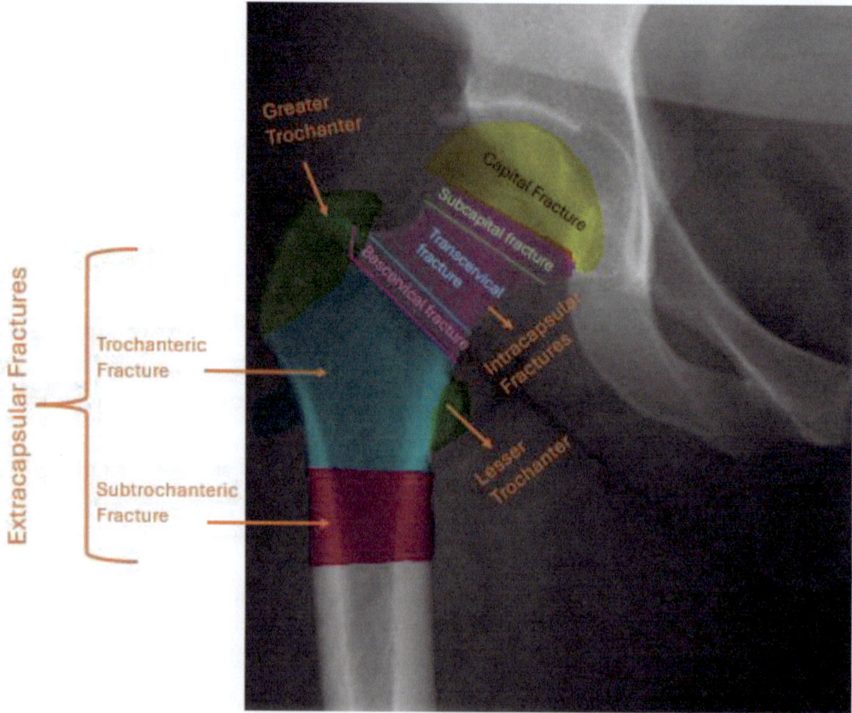

Fig. 14.1 Types of femur pathologies

14.3.2 Subcapital Fracture

This is an intracapsular fracture that occurs below the head of the femur, at the junction between the head and neck of the femur (*see* Fig. 14.2).

14.3.3 Basicervical

This is an intracapsular fracture seen at the base of the femoral neck, close to the intertrochanteric line. It lies between the femoral neck and the intertrochanteric region (*see* Fig. 14.3).

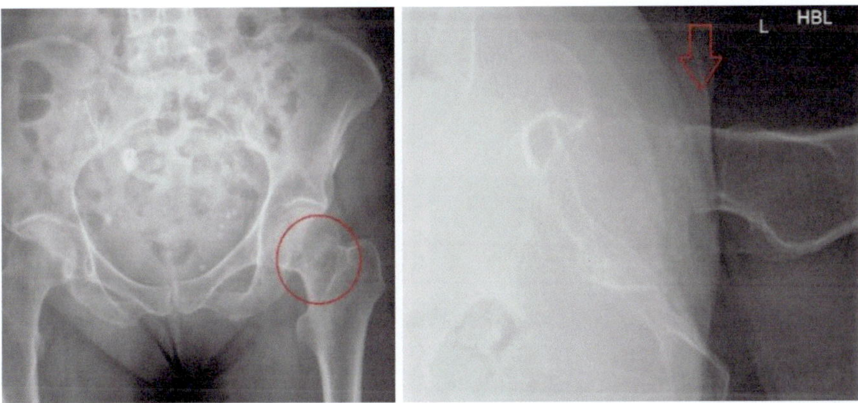

Fig. 14.2 Subcapital fracture

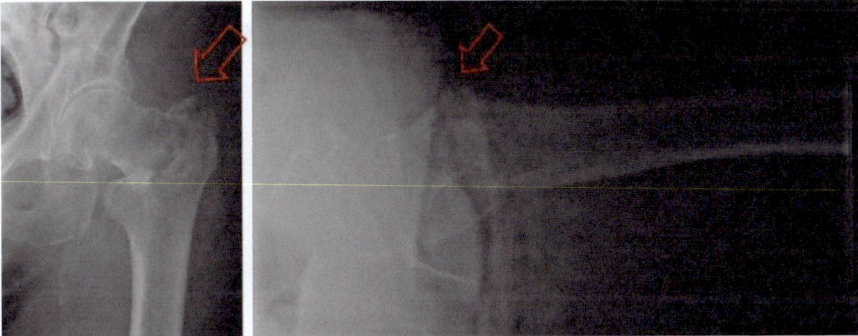

Fig. 14.3 Basicervical fracture

14.3.4 Transcervical

This is an intracapsular fracture that occurs through the mid-portion of the femoral neck, between the head of the femur and the intertrochanteric line (*see* Fig. 14.4).

14.3.5 Intertrochanteric

This is an extracapsular fracture of the proximal femur that occurs through the lesser and greater trochanter (*see* Fig. 14.5).

14.3.6 Subtrochanteric

This is an extracapsular fracture that occurs in the proximal third of the femoral shaft, just below the lesser trochanter. It is commonly seen as a transverse fracture (*see* Fig. 14.6).

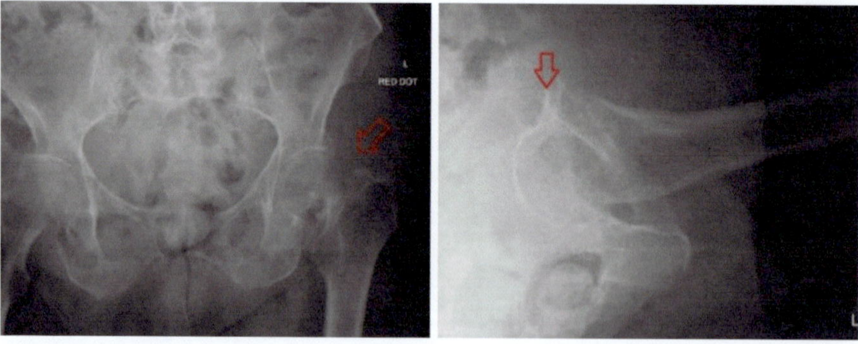

Fig. 14.4 Transcervical fracture

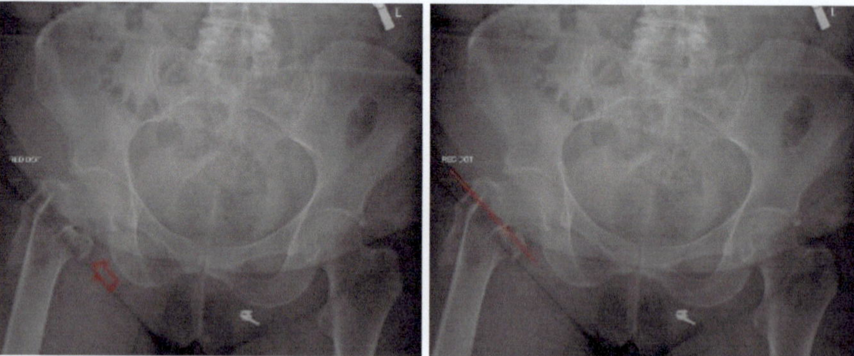

Fig. 14.5 Intertrochanteric fracture

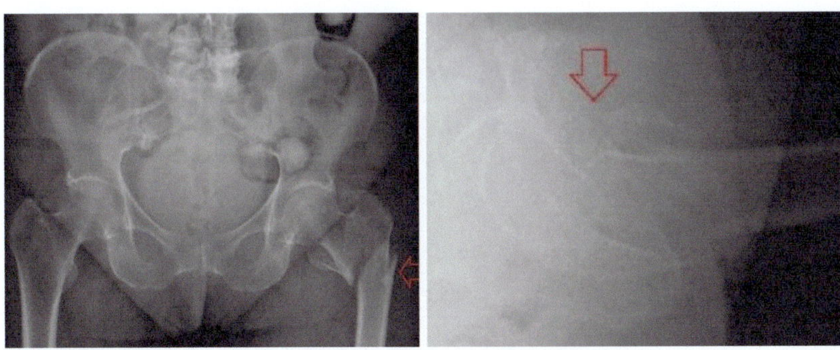

Fig. 14.6 Subtrochanteric fracture

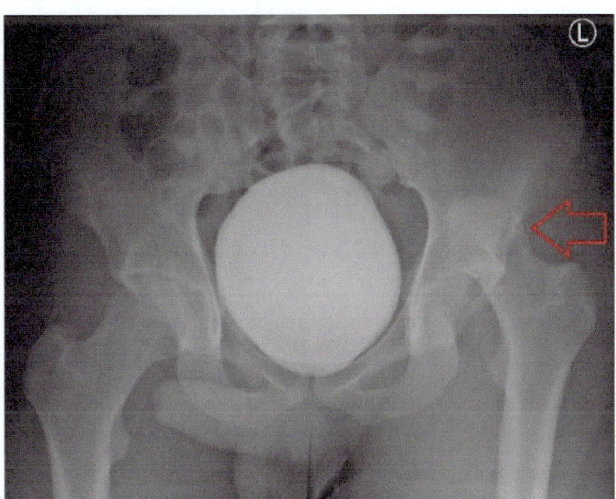

Fig. 14.7 Anterior femoral dislocation

14.3.7 Anterior Femoral Dislocation

This occurs when the head of the femur is displaced anteriorly, causing it to be visible in front of the acetabulum.

Figure 14.7 shows the femur to be anteriorly displaced, with the femur lying in front of the acetabulum, but also superiorly, as it is seen above the acetabular region.

14.3.8 Posterior Femoral Dislocation

This occurs when the head of the femur is displaced posteriorly, causing it to be visible behind the acetabulum (*see* Fig. 14.8).

Fig. 14.8 Posterior femoral fracture

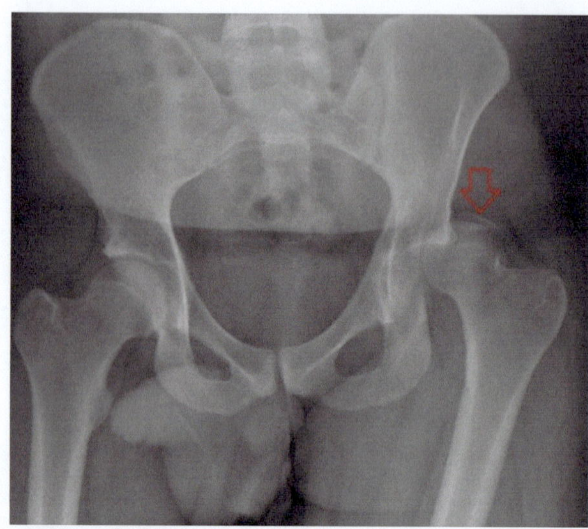

Fig. 14.9 Greater trochanteric fracture

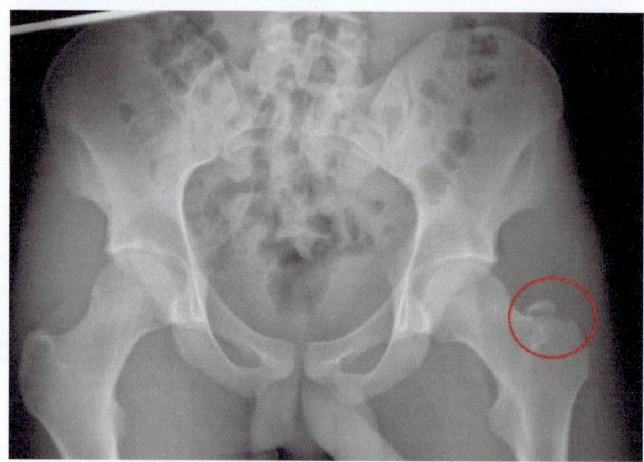

14.3.9 Greater Trochanter Fracture

A greater trochanter fracture involves the lateral bony prominence of the proximal femur (*see* Fig. 14.9). It may occur in isolation or alongside intertrochanteric or femoral neck fractures.

Fig. 14.10 Lesser trochanteric fracture

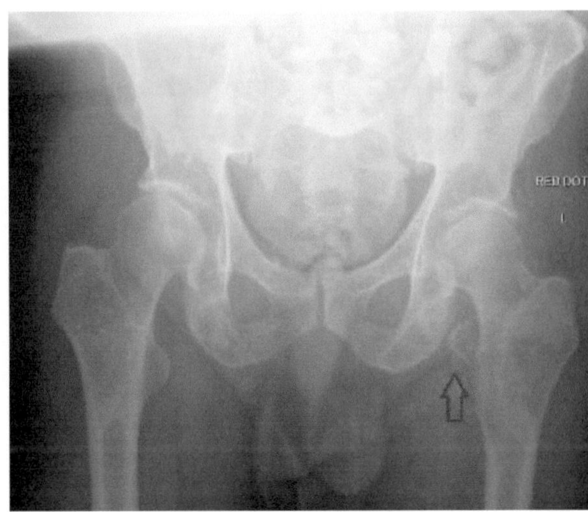

14.3.10 Lesser Trochanter Fracture

A lesser trochanter fracture involves a break at the bony prominence on the medial aspect of the proximal femur (*see* Fig. 14.10). These fractures are often seen in association with other proximal femoral injuries and may be displaced due to the pull of the iliopsoas muscle. Isolated fractures of the lesser trochanter are rare and, especially in adults, may suggest underlying metastatic disease.

References

1. Whitley AS, Jefferson G, Holmes K, Sloane C, Anderson C. Clark's positioning in radiography. 13th ed. CRC Press; 2015.
2. Greenspan A. Orthopedic imaging: a practical approach. 6th ed. Wolters Kluwer; 2015.

Figure 15.1 demonstrates the basic anatomical structures visible on a standard anteroposterior (AP) pelvic x-ray.

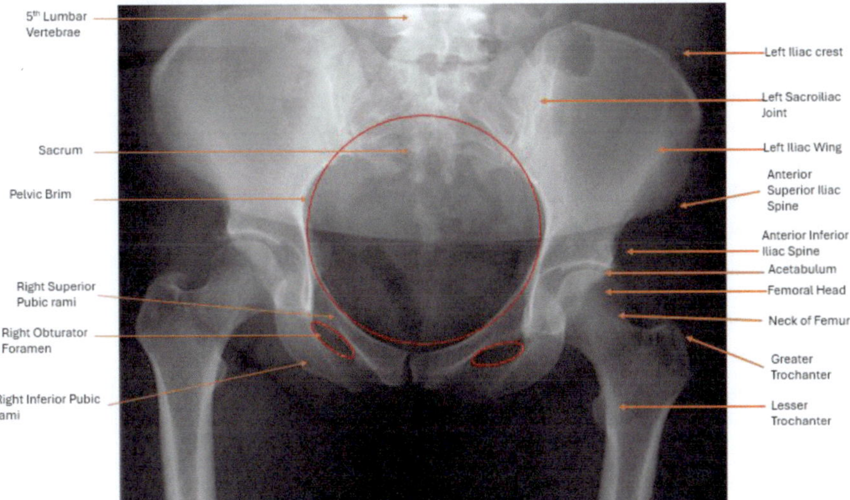

Fig. 15.1 Anatomical structures of the pelvis on the AP view

S. Moughal, *Fracture Finder: A Practical Guide to Interpreting Upper and Lower Limb X-Rays for Radiographers*,
https://doi.org/10.1007/978-3-032-17324-9_15

15.1   Standard Views, Centring Points and Area of Interest

Anteroposterior   The pelvis is centred to the image receptor. Both legs are internally rotated 15–20 degrees to align the femoral necks parallel to the receptor. The central ray is directed to the point midway between the anterior superior iliac spines (ASIS) and the pubic symphysis. Figure 15.1 shows the entire pelvis from the iliac crests to the proximal femora.

Area of Interest   The image should include the entire pelvis from the iliac crests down to the proximal femora, and both hip joints should be visible. Ensure the femoral necks are well seen without foreshortening. The pubic symphysis and acetabula must be included to assess for fractures or dislocations.

15.2   General Evaluation of Pelvis Examinations

1. The image should include the entire pelvis, from the iliac crests superiorly to below the ischial tuberosities inferiorly, and extend laterally to include both hip joints.
2. The pelvis should be well centred on the image receptor, with correct collimation to include all relevant anatomy and reduce patient dose.
3. Bony cortices and trabecular patterns should be clearly defined, with no motion blur or artefacts.
4. Assess the sacroiliac joints, pubic symphysis and acetabula for alignment, joint space narrowing or widening.
5. Check for fractures, cortical irregularities or signs of pelvic ring disruption.
6. Both proximal femora should be included and examined for possible associated injury.
7. Evaluate the soft tissues for signs of swelling, haematoma or gas.
8. The image should be free from rotation or positioning errors, ensuring accurate visualisation of pelvic symmetry and joint alignment [1].

When evaluating the pelvis, several key lines must be assessed (*see* Fig. 15.2) to ensure there are no hidden pathologies. Disruption of any of these lines could indicate the presence of a fracture.

These lines are:

- Shenton's line: This is a smooth curve that connects the inferior border of the superior pubic ramus to the inner edge of the neck of femur.
- Posterior acetabular line: The curved line formed by the posterior wall of the acetabulum, normally seen just behind the femoral head.
- Roof of the acetabulum: This lines the superior aspect of the acetabulum, which is seen just above the femoral head.
- Teardrop: This is a teardrop-shaped outline which is formed by the medial wall of the acetabulum and the acetabular floor.

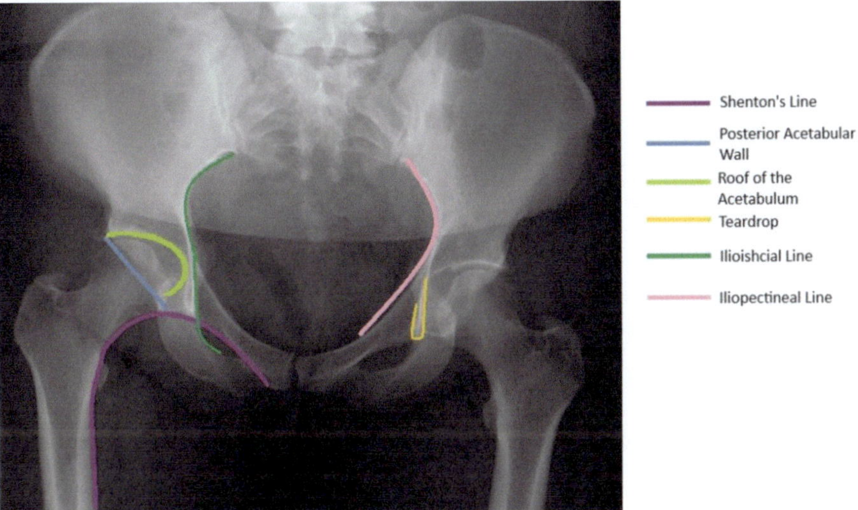

Fig. 15.2 Lines to assess when checking pelvic x-rays

- Ilioischial line: this is a smooth line seen following the posterior column of the acetabulum, running from the ilium to the ischium.
- Iliopectineal line: This is a smooth line on pelvic X-rays that follows the anterior column of the acetabulum, running from the ilium to the pubis.

Must check the three pelvic rings if one of them is disrupted, then there is a possibility of more than one fracture.

Much check joint spaces—must be symmetrical—SIJ (should be 2-4 mm)— symph (no more than 5 mm) Assess acetabulum.

15.3 Common Pelvic Fracture/Pathologies

15.3.1 Acetabular Fracture

This is a fracture of the socket part of the hip joint, known as the acetabulum (*see* Fig. 15.3). It is where the head of the femur articulates with the pelvis.

Fig. 15.3 Acetabular
fracture

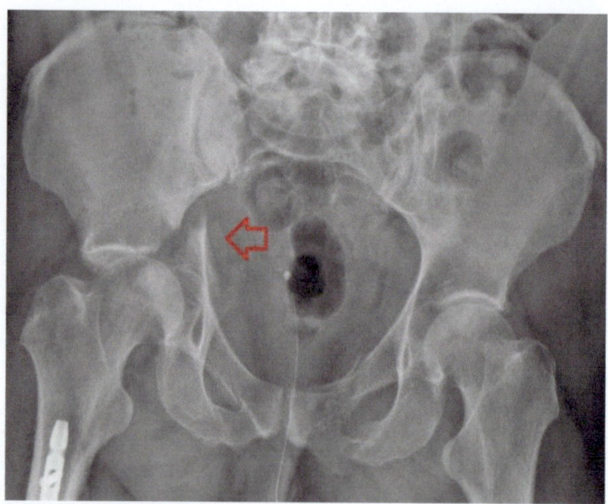

Fig. 15.4 Avulsion
fracture of the AIIS

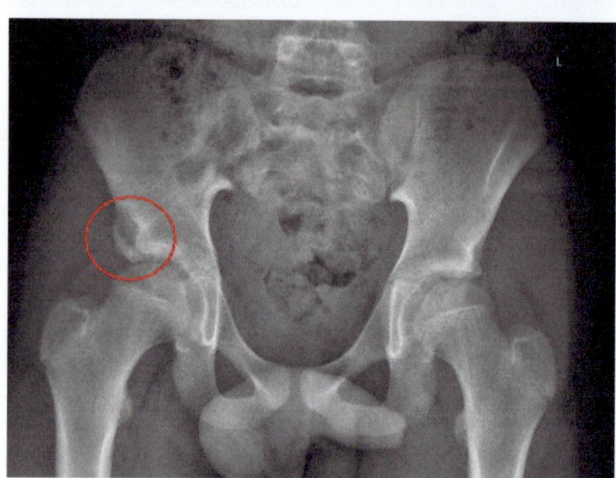

15.3.2 Avulsion of the ASIS/AIIS

This occurs when a small piece of bone is pulled off (avulsed), making it an avulsion fracture of the anterior superior iliac spine (ASIS). Similar avulsion fractures can also happen at the anterior inferior iliac spine (AIIS) or the ischial tuberosity (*see* Fig. 15.4).

15.3.3 Duverney

This is a fracture seen through the iliac wing of the pelvis (*see* Fig. 15.5).

Fig. 15.5 Duverney fracture

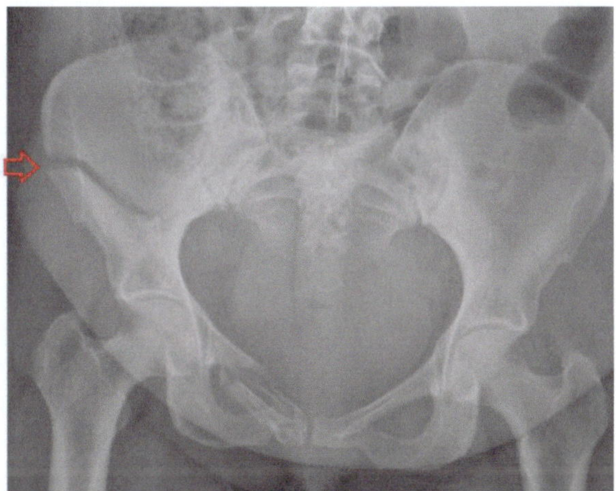

Fig. 15.6 Ishiopubic rami fracture

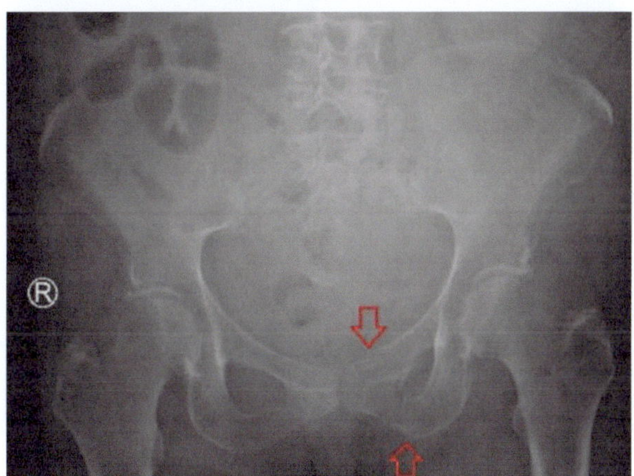

15.3.4 Sacral Fracture

This is typically a longitudinal fracture going through the sacrum.

15.3.5 Ischiopubic Rami Fracture

This is a fracture involving the ischium and pubic rami. It can be unilateral, affecting one pubic ramus, or bilateral, involving both pubic rami.

Fig. 15.6 shows a fracture going through both superior and inferior pubic rami on the left side.

15.3.6 Malgaigne

This is a type of pelvic fracture involving a vertical fracture of the ipsilateral (same side) superior and inferior pubic rami combined with a disruption of the sacroiliac joint or sacral fracture on the same side (*see* Fig. 15.7).

15.3.7 Straddle

This is a bilateral fracture of the superior and inferior pubic rami, involving both obturator foramen rings (*see* Fig. 15.8). It usually results from high-energy trauma and can cause pelvic instability.

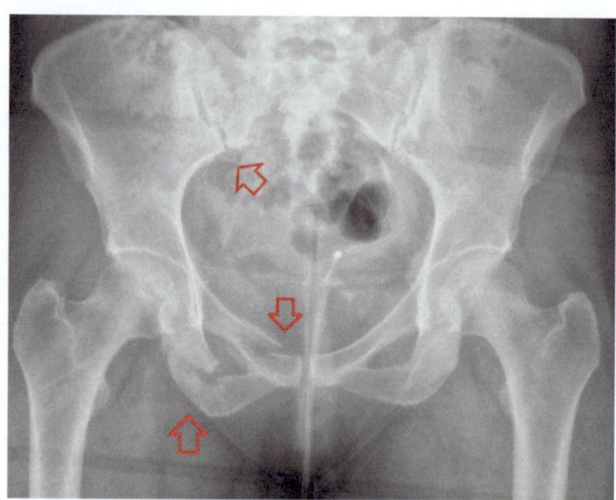

Fig. 15.7 Malgaigne fracture

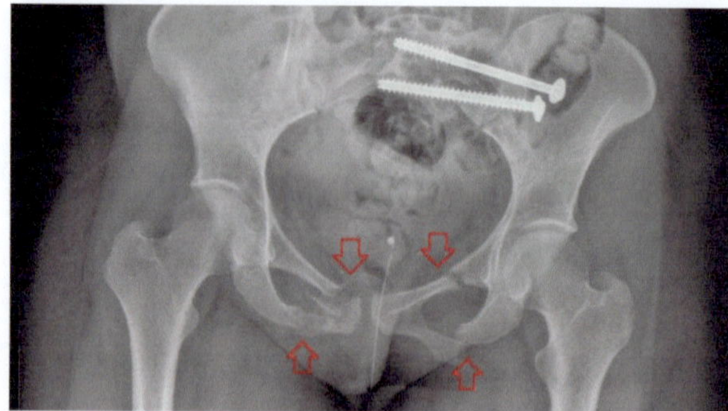

Fig. 15.8 Straddle fracture

15.3.8 Bucket Handle

This is a vertically orientated fracture through the ipsilateral (same side) superior and inferior pubic rami with contralateral (opposite side) Sacro-iliac joint dislocation or disruption (*see* Fig. 15.9).

15.3.9 Sprung

This is when both sacroiliac joints are dislocated and there is widening of the pubic symphysis (*see* Fig. 15.10).

Fig. 15.9 Bucket-handle injury

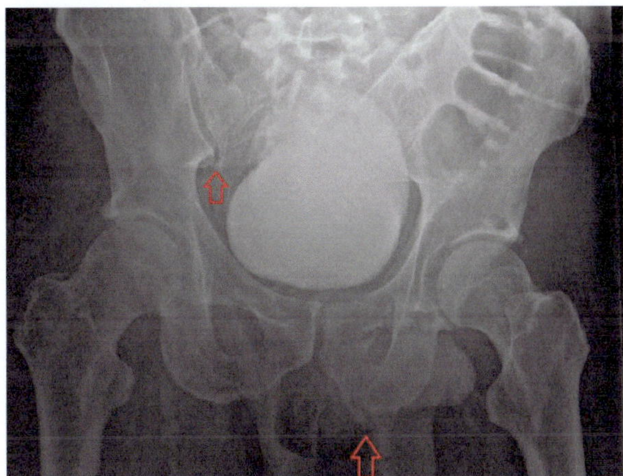

Fig. 15.10 Sprung injury

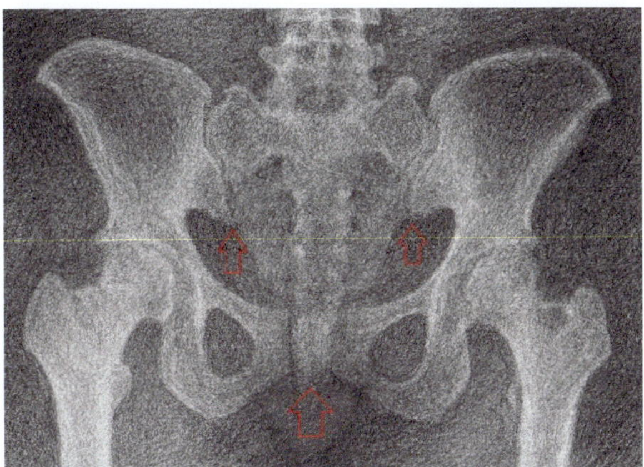

Fig. 15.11 Open book injury

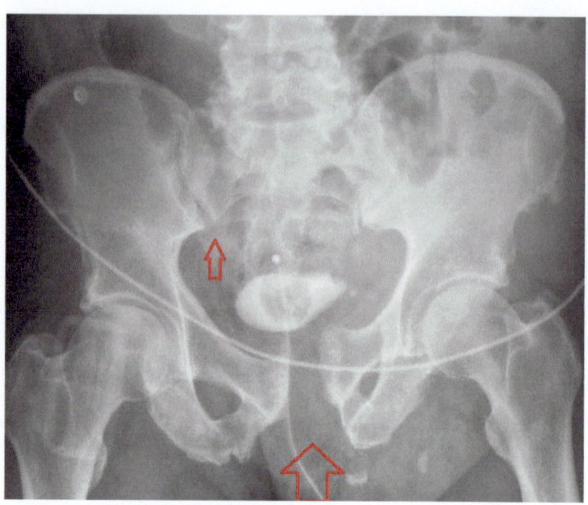

15.3.10 Open Book

This is a pelvic fracture where the pubic symphysis is widened and one of the sacroiliac joints is dislocated (*see* Fig. 15.11).

Reference

1. Carver E, Carver B. Medical imaging: techniques, reflection & evaluation. 2nd ed. Wiley-Blackwell; 2012.

Glossary

Acetabulum The cup-shaped socket of the hip bone that articulates with the femoral head.

Alignment The correct positioning of body parts and X-ray beam to ensure accurate imaging and diagnosis.

Angulation The angle formed between bone fragments at a fracture site or the tilt of the X-ray tube.

Anteroposterior (AP) View A projection where the X-ray beam travels from the front (anterior) to the back (posterior).

Area of Interest (AOI) The specific anatomical region that must be fully included in an image for accurate diagnosis.

Avulsion Fracture A fracture where a fragment of bone is pulled away by a tendon or ligament.

Bennett's Fracture An intra-articular fracture at the base of the first metacarpal extending into the carpometacarpal joint.

Bimalleolar Fracture Fracture involving both the medial and lateral malleoli of the ankle.

Bohr's Angle The angle between the anterior and posterior borders of the calcaneus; decreased in calcaneal fracture.

Boxer's Fracture A fracture at the neck of the fifth metacarpal, typically caused by punching.

Bone Trabeculae The fine network of bone tissue visible within cancellous bone on X-ray.

Callus Formation New bone growth seen around a healing fracture.

Capitellar Line A line drawn through the centre of the radial neck that should pass through the capitellum; used to assess elbow alignment.

Carpometacarpal (CMC) Joint The joint between the distal carpal bones and the metacarpals of the hand.

Centring Point The precise anatomical location at which the X-ray beam is aimed.

Colles' Fracture Extra-articular distal radius fracture with posterior displacement of the distal fragment.

© The Editor(s) (if applicable) and The Author(s), under exclusive license to Springer Nature Switzerland AG 2026

S. Moughal, *Fracture Finder: A Practical Guide to Interpreting Upper and Lower Limb X-Rays for Radiographers*, https://doi.org/10.1007/978-3-032-17324-9

Collimation Restricting the X-ray beam to the area of interest to minimise patient dose and scatter.

Comminuted Fracture A fracture where the bone is broken into three or more fragments.

Contrast The visible difference in density between adjacent areas on an X-ray image.

Displacement Movement of bone fragments from their normal anatomical position.

Distal Away from the centre of the body or the point of attachment.

Dorsoplantar (DP) View Projection of the foot from the dorsal (top) to the plantar (bottom) surface.

Duverney Fracture A fracture through the iliac wing of the pelvis.

Epiphysis The end section of a long bone that ossifies separately from the shaft.

Exposure Factors Technical settings (kVp, mAs, SID) used to produce an X-ray image of diagnostic quality.

Extension Straightening movement increasing the angle between two bones.

Fat Pad Sign Elevation of the elbow joint's fat pad, suggesting joint effusion and possible occult fracture.

Field of View (FOV) The anatomical region included in the radiographic image.

Fracture Line A visible break or crack in bone continuity.

Galeazzi Fracture Fracture of the distal or midshaft radius with dislocation of the distal radioulnar joint.

Greenstick Fracture Incomplete fracture in children where one side of the bone bends, while the other breaks.

Grid A device used to reduce scatter radiation and improve image contrast.

Hallux Valgus Lateral deviation of the great toe with medial deviation of the first metatarsal.

Hill-Sachs Lesion A compression fracture on the posterolateral humeral head due to anterior shoulder dislocation.

Horizontal Beam X-ray beam parallel to the floor, often used in trauma imaging.

Humeroglenoid Dislocation Displacement of the humeral head from the glenoid fossa, either anteriorly or posteriorly.

Impacted Fracture Fracture where bone fragments are driven into each other.

Internal Rotation Turning of a limb toward the body's midline.

Intra-articular Fracture A fracture extending into a joint space.

Jones Fracture Transverse fracture of the fifth metatarsal at the metaphyseal-diaphyseal junction.

Joint Space The visible gap between articulating bones on an image; irregularity may indicate pathology.

Knee Joint Space The gap between the femur and tibia; narrowing suggests degenerative change.

Lateral View An X-ray taken from the side of a body part.

Lisfranc Injury Fracture dislocation of the tarsometatarsal joints of the foot.

Lucent An area appearing darker on an image due to reduced density (e.g., air, soft tissue).

Mallet Finger Flexion deformity of the distal phalanx due to avulsion of the extensor tendon.

Maisonneuve Fracture Proximal fibular fracture with associated medial malleolar injury.

Medial Towards the midline of the body.

Monteggia Fracture Fracture of the proximal ulna with dislocation of the radial head.

Mortise View 15–20° internally rotated AP ankle view showing the ankle joint space clearly.

Oblique View Projection taken at an angle between AP and lateral positions.

Osgood–Schlatter Disease Inflammation of the tibial tuberosity due to stress at the patellar ligament attachment.

Open Fracture Fracture where the bone penetrates the skin.

Pathology Abnormality or disease process visible on an image.

Patella Alta Abnormally high-riding patella, often indicating tendon disruption.

Periosteum A thin fibrous membrane covering the bone surface.

Positioning Patient and limb alignment used to produce optimal diagnostic images.

Posterior Referring to the back surface of the body or structure.

Projection The path of the X-ray beam through the body.

Radiolucent Permitting X-rays to pass through; appears dark on an image.

Radiopaque Blocking X-rays; appears light or white on an image.

Region of Interest (ROI) The specific anatomical region to be examined.

Rotation Turning of a body part around its long axis.

Salter-Harris Classification System describing fractures involving the growth plate in paediatric patients (Types I–V).

Scaphoid Fracture Fracture through the waist or poles of the scaphoid bone; risk of avascular necrosis proximally.

Segond Fracture Small avulsion fracture of the lateral tibial plateau, often associated with ACL injury.

Shenton's Line Smooth curve formed by the superior border of the obturator foramen and femoral neck; disruption suggests hip fracture.

SID (Source-to-Image Distance) Distance between the X-ray tube and image receptor.

Smith's Fracture Extra-articular distal radius fracture with anterior displacement of the distal fragment.

Soft Tissue Shadow Radiographic outline of soft tissue, helpful for identifying swelling or foreign bodies.

Subluxation Partial dislocation of a joint.

Supination Outward rotation of the forearm or foot.

Teardrop Sign Normal radiographic feature of the acetabulum; disruption may suggest pelvic fracture.

Torus (Buckle) Fracture Incomplete compression fracture commonly seen in paediatric patients.

Transverse Fracture A fracture with a horizontal line perpendicular to the long axis of the bone.

Trimalleolar Fracture Fracture involving the medial, lateral and posterior malleoli.

Ulnar Deviation Movement of the wrist towards the ulna (little finger side).

Undisplaced Fracture Fracture where the bone fragments remain in anatomical alignment.

View The radiographic image corresponding to a specific projection.

Volar Relating to the palmar or plantar surface (front of hand or sole of foot).

Volar Plate Avulsion Fracture Avulsion of the palmar aspect of the base of the middle phalanx, typically from hyperextension.

Weight-Bearing View Image taken while the patient is standing to evaluate joint alignment under load.

®
FSC
www.fsc.org
MIX
Papier aus verantwortungsvollen Quellen
Paper from responsible sources
FSC® C105338